Change Your Life!

SIMPLE STRATEGIES TO LOSE WEIGHT, GET FIT AND IMPROVE YOUR OUTLOOK

D1411372

Change Your Life!

SIMPLE STRATEGIES TO LOSE WEIGHT, GET FIT AND IMPROVE YOUR OUTLOOK

An official publication of the

Arthritis Foundation

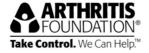

Change Your Life!

Simple Strategies To Lose Weight,
Get Fit and Improve Your Outlook

Published by the Arthritis Foundation
1330 West Peachtree Street
Atlanta, GA 30309

800/283-7800
www.arthritis.org

Printed in Canada
1st Printing 2002

Library of Congress Card Catalog Number:
2002100856

ISBN: 0-912423-30-7

CONTENTS

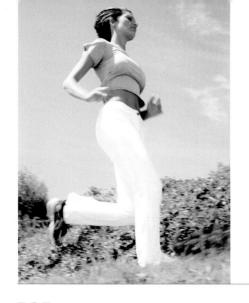

[2] Why Should You Change?

If you didn't need to make some changes, you wouldn't have picked up this book. So we'll begin by working through your barriers to change and reinforcing why change is so important.

[12] The Road to Change: Where Are You Now?

What's the first step in moving toward a healthier future? Understanding where you stand today.

[30] Celebrate Your Success Smartly and Stay Motivated

Positive first steps are a great way to start. But you will only achieve success through sustained change. Staying motivated with the following tips will help you reach that goal.

[40] Change the Way You Eat

Making small changes to what you eat every day and what you keep in your pantry can help you cut calories and fat gradually. That's the best way to keep excess calories out of your life for good!

[70] Change the Way You Think About Exercise

Exercise can help you burn more calories, lose weight and keep it off, feel more energetic and be more flexible. So why do so many people hate to do it? Here are some simple strategies to get limber, fit and strong.

[104] Change Your Outlook

Improving the way you handle stress can make it easier for you to attain all of your other change-your-life goals.

[120] Now Is The Time To Change Your Life

Now that you've learned the three aspects of change and some great techniques for making permanent, positive change, get going!

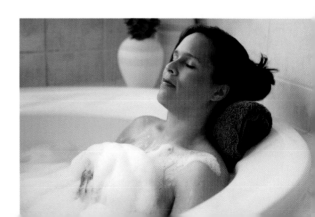

Acknowledgements

Change Your Life: Simple Strategies to Lose Weight, Get Fit and Improve Your Outlook is the proud result of a yearlong cooperative effort between the editors of *Arthritis Today* magazine, staff of the Arthritis Foundation and several dedicated Arthritis Foundation volunteers and health-care professionals. The book is based on the series *Arthritis Today's You First Challenge,* which ran in each issue of *Arthritis Today* in 2001. The series focused on empowering readers to make positive changes to diet, fitness, outlook and general health practices.

Many *Arthritis Today* writers, editors and staff members contributed to this series and to the elements of the series that are included in this book: Marcy O'Koon Moss, Editor and Associate Vice President; Audrey Graham, Art Director; Beth Blaney, Managing Editor; Stacy Baker, Senior Editor; Michele Taylor, Associate Editor; Kaetrena Davis, Publishing Assistant; and Melanie Lasoff, Contributing Editor.

In addition, acknowledgements should go to the following Arthritis Foundation staff members who created this book: Susan Bernstein, Director, Book Development and Acquisition, who wrote the text of the book; Susan Siracusa, Associate Art Director, Publishing, who designed the interior and the cover of the book; and Katie Culley Kroll, Manager, Custom Publishing, who contributed to the book's editing and development. Members of the Arthritis Foundation's Programs and Services department also served as advisors to the development of the book, including Shannon Whetstone Mescher, M.Ed.,CHES, and Linda Spence, MS. Special thanks also to Suzanne Verity, Associate Vice President, Custom Publishing, for her guidance and support during the writing of this book.

The medical editor of this book was John H. Klippel, MD, Medical Director of the Arthritis Foundation. Also assisting with the development of this book were volunteers Nancy Anderson, RD; Patricia Grosklaus, PT; and Dorothy Leone-Glasser, RN.

READY
SET
GO!

A note from *Arthritis Today* Editor
Marcy O'Koon Moss:

It's time for a new you. No matter where you are in your pursuit of better health and a more positive outlook, you can start now by eating better, exercising more and just plain taking care of yourself. By picking up this book, you have taken the first step. This book can help. As you change your life, all the editors and health professionals who developed *Change Your Life* will be there for you, motivating you, educating you – and showing you just how doable this health-improvement plan can be.

This is about putting you first. Why should you put you first? That's selfish, you say? We beg to differ. When you are in less pain and have more energy, more range of motion and a better outlook on life, then you have more to give others.

Putting you first really means taking care of yourself. It means making movement a part of your life again. It means eating right. And it means maintaining emotional health, too – saying goodbye to stress, improving relationships and feeling hopeful.

Together, let's begin this journey of discovery and challenge. This process is all about getting to know yourself. What will it take for you to put yourself first? Some of us are more ready than others for this life-change. Are you skeptical or are you sold? Doesn't matter. Wherever you are on this journey, the steps are yours to take. One person might need the courage to take her first walk around the block; another may need the conviction to stop his on-again off-again pattern of exercise; yet another may need kudos to recognize just how well she's doing and the encouragement to take it up a notch.

You might try sharing this book or the strategies contained in these pages with your husband or wife, your sister or brother, a neighbor or a friend. You can motivate each other, a great way to keep yourself focused and moving forward. If we stick together, we'll all make progress, but we may not end up in the same place, because we didn't all start in the same place. You need to succeed on your own terms, at your own pace. Don't compare your success to another person's success – every person is unique.

Ready? OK, then. The first two chapters focus on self-assessment. Think of it as the "You Are Here" arrow on a map. In every chapter, we'll look at ways you can get more exercise, eat better, lose weight (even 10 pounds can make a big difference in how you feel), improve your outlook and let the sun shine in.

Are you ready to change your life?

Great! Here we go!

IS IT TIME To Change?

Change Your Life...We can hear you respond to this call to action right now: "Oh, yeah? Why should I change my life?"

If everything in your life – your weight, your fitness or stress level, your overall sense of well-being – is in perfect order, then maybe you shouldn't change a thing. But...does that sound like your life?

Take a quick inventory of your life – or, more specifically, your health and your lifestyle. Is your weight a little bit more than you would like it to be, or significantly greater than it should be? Do you exercise once a week, once a month or never at all? Do you get stressed out only occasionally, when work or family pressures become too intense? Or do you find that you become tense and upset at the slightest problem, from a broken traffic light to your son dropping an ice cream bar on the kitchen floor?

So...why should you change your life? Why should you make changing your diet a priority, or make time for exercise, or find ways to relax your body and mind at the end of a tough day?

Because you owe it to yourself to put you first. That's a tough order for many people. Kids, job, husbands and wives, parents, household chores and bills – those obligations come first. But yourself? Where do you place yourself – your health, your happiness, your well-being, your emotional outlook – on the scale of important things in your life? It's time to take stock of how you are doing, how you are feeling and what you need in order to succeed at your goals. As this book's title suggests, in these pages we will show you some simple strategies to accomplish a few, all-important goals: losing weight, increasing fitness and reducing or controlling stress. We also will show you how to assess where you stand in your overall health and fitness, and how you can track your success.

The information in this book is based on a year-long series in *Arthritis Today* magazine called *Arthritis Today's* "You First Challenge." In this challenge, readers learned simple techniques for making positive changes to their diet, fitness level and outlook on life. They are encouraged to set goals and track progress.

Change Your Life builds on and adds to some of the strategies presented in *Arthritis Today* to give you a handy, comprehensive and life-changing guidebook. *Change Your Life* can be used by anyone who wishes to make positive adjustments to their health, fitness and emotional well-being. While you don't have to have arthritis to use the strategies outlined here, it's important to note that many common health conditions, including arthritis, can be helped through sensible weight loss, exercise and stress-control techniques.

Along with effective medications and surgery, many doctors prescribe a healthy diet, regular exercise and stress control to their patients dealing with many health problems, including heart disease, osteoarthritis, diabetes and more.

This book will help you explore some of the aspects of diet and nutrition, fitness and stress control. You'll learn ways to control your calorie intake with tasty, nutritious foods, and how to burn calories through doable exercises.

[*You will discover the power of positive change as you read and use* Change Your Life.]

But your doctor is the best source of information when it comes to your health. This book gives you helpful resources, positive suggestions and encouragement for you as you begin your quest to change your life. Consult your doctor or other health-care professional before changing your normal routine. You and your doctor can work together to determine what types of changes are best for you, according to your personal health status and physical abilities.

Change Your Life is a great place to start your quest to achieve better health. You are embarking on an exciting, beneficial and, perhaps, challenging journey. With this book as your guide, get ready to take the first step on that journey now – it's time to put one foot forward and change your life!

WHY Should You CHANGE?

If you didn't need to make some changes, you wouldn't have picked up this book. So we'll begin by working through your barriers to change and reinforcing why change is so important.

Most people don't like to change. They would like to see changes in the reading on the bathroom scale, or how their stomach looks in a sweater. But changing from eating fried potatoes to a plain baked potato, or altering your after-work routine from sitting in front of the TV to taking a brisk walk? That kind of change seems daunting, difficult and, for some people, depressing.

Unfortunately, there is no easy way to make yourself healthier and more fit if you are not in that state now. Despite the seemingly magical claims of many products advertised on TV,

[*"Why should I change my life? Isn't there an easier way?"*]

products that claim you can drink a concoction or take a pill to melt fat away, most health ex-

perts say that having a healthy body requires some effort on your part. Not an extreme effort – people who try to make extreme changes often fail and wind up worse off than before – but a gradual, moderate effort to change bad habits into healthy ones. The goal is to get in better shape – both physically and emotionally.

When your body and emotions are out of shape, you may find it more difficult to handle the important tasks in your life, from your job to your relationships. You might find it more difficult to do enjoyable activities too, like sailing with friends at the lake or taking your mother bargain-hunting at garage sales early Saturday morning.

There is a vicious cycle at work here – you might have more energy and desire to do more for yourself and your loved ones if you could only lose weight, get in shape or feel better. If

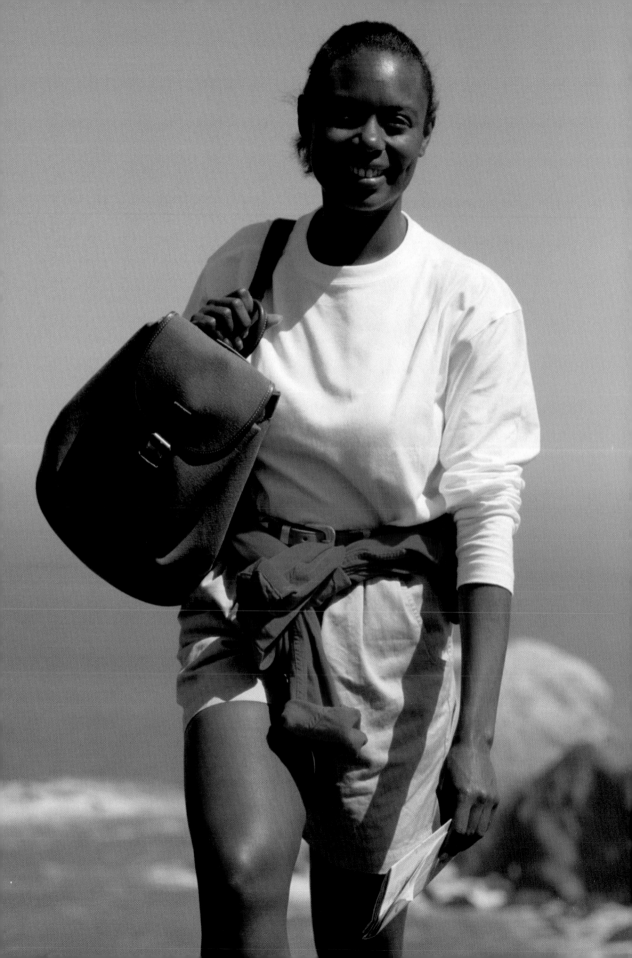

you feel sluggish and tired every morning, and worse every evening after a full day at work or at home with the kids, where will you find the energy to go to a movie or a school play?

In your mind, you may have an image of yourself as a few pounds thinner, more physically fit, with more energy to do more enjoyable activities. It's a goal that seems so real, yet at times, so unattainable. Accomplishing that all-important goal – the goal of positive personal change – is daunting for many people. At times, it seems impossible. So why even try?

Because you are worth it. You are worth just one more try.

Change – A Gradual Process

Changing your life, and putting yourself first, isn't something you can do all at once. Forget that idea right this second. This kind of change takes time. You must accept that fact – you can change, and if you really want to change, you *will* change. Slowly, you can make small changes in your diet, your activity and your emotional health that will all come together to create a big positive change in you.

Along the road to change, you'll probably stumble a few times. You may have to take two steps backward in order to take one step forward. That's OK! As long as you make some progress in the long run, you have accomplished something. You need to congratulate yourself, celebrating everyday victories rather than just giant triumphs. You will learn how to identify everyday victories and ways to celebrate them right here in this book. You'll discover that simple, positive choices – such as taking the stairs to your third floor office instead of riding in the elevator – can be "everyday victories." You'll find that it's OK to celebrate making this choice, and

to congratulate yourself for taking positive steps in the name of change.

RESOLUTIONS – EASY TO MAKE, EASY TO BREAK

Each January, nearly everyone makes "New Year's resolutions" in which they pledge to change their diet, quit smoking or exercise every day after work. Weight loss programs and gyms are more crowded than at any other time of the year, filled with well-meaning men and women who have lofty self-improvement goals – "If I can just do this for six months, I know I can lose 20 pounds. I know I can fit into that outfit for my sister's wedding."

Does this scenario sound familiar? Probably so.

Most people set life-changing goals at one time or another. Perhaps you have tried to lose weight to fit into a certain outfit or to look your best for a wedding or your high school reunion. You might resolve to go on a weight-loss program on New Year's Day, after spending the evening before drinking champagne and the morning after watching football games over a plate of nachos. Weight-loss programs are crowded in January, but often dwindle in size by March.

It isn't that people don't want to change – it's just that change is hard to sustain. It can seem impossible. Resolutions are easy to make and easy to break. "Well, I tried to keep my eating under control, but I just like to eat at the pizza parlor with the guys after work. I like to be able to eat as much pizza as I want without thinking about 'portion control.' Boring! I don't want to. So what? I guess I can try again later."

So what happens when we break the good habits we pledged to keep back on January 1? Maybe we're in a slump for a while, reverting to old habits of overeating high-fat foods, smoking cigarettes or sitting on the couch instead of taking a short walk after work. But after a while, something spurs us to try again, perhaps another special family event, or a frustrating trip to the mall to try on pairs of pants that seem tight and uncomfortable. We start over, trying to change our habits again and again and again, only to go right back where we were before.

It's easy to get discouraged. At times, you might say, "It isn't worth it. I will always be this way. I just have to come to grips with that fact. I will always be overweight, and I will never exercise regularly, and I will just have to deal with it. I will never change. What will be will be."

CHANGE NOW – OR REGRET IT LATER?

If you don't change unhealthy habits, can there be serious consequences? The answer is yes.

According to the National Institutes of Health (NIH), being overweight can increase your risk of diabetes, heart disease, stroke, hypertension (high blood pressure), gallbladder disease, osteoarthritis, some forms of cancer, and sleep apnea or other breathing problems. Not a pleasant prospect!

Unfortunately, despite the large amounts of information on nutrition and the explosion of lower-fat and lower-calorie foods on the market, more and more Americans are overweight or obese. This means that the person has an abnormally high proportion of body fat, according to body fat-measurement tests. According to the NIH, more than half of U.S. adults are overweight, and nearly one quarter of Americans are not only overweight, but obese.

In addition, the percentage of adults who are overweight has increased steadily in recent years. Ironically, people seem to want to lose this excess weight very badly. Government re-

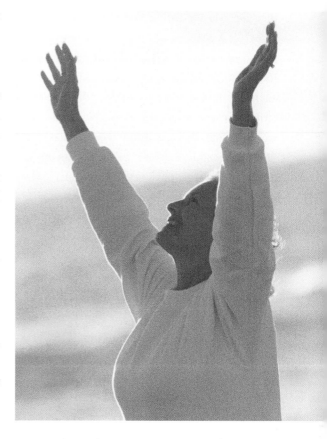

ports show that Americans spend $33 billion annually on weight-loss products and services. However, when you compare this statistic with the statistics about so many Americans being overweight, it is apparent that something isn't working. People try various weight-loss programs or products, lose weight in the short term, but then gain the weight they lost right back. Sometimes, they gain back more pounds than they lost in the first place.

While people may want to lose weight, they find it hard to maintain the changes they make in their diets. So they give up. It happens all the time. This unfortunate cycle of weight loss and weight gain leads many people to become discouraged. Why do they struggle to maintain the healthy changes that helped them lose weight? Because most people try to drastically change their lifestyle and eating habits. They feel that a "diet" or a weight-loss program is a temporary period of austerity, when they eat all the right foods and do all the right things to stay fit. The change is drastic, but they feel that they are suffering for the short term so they can lose weight. Once they have lost weight, they feel that they don't have to eat healthfully anymore. Old habits return, and so do the pounds.

Hopefully, this book will illustrate ways that you can change gradually, so that you will be better able to keep those changes in your routine. By slowly introducing small changes into your routine, you will become used to eating in a new way and incorporating exercise into your daily life. It won't seem like a drastic change. But the change that you see in yourself will be powerful in the long run.

When it comes to physical activity, another key factor in reducing the risk of developing some diseases and a great way to lose excess weight, the statistics are no more encouraging. According to the NIH, only 22 percent of U.S. adults get the recommended amount of physical activity – at least 30 minutes of physical activity at least five times a week. About one quarter of U.S. adults say they do no physical activity in their leisure time. It's not surprising that so many Americans are overweight and dealing with difficult health problems.

Exercise not only helps you control your weight, it can boost your energy levels so you can enjoy your activities more. Being in good physical shape improves your appearance, boosts your self-esteem, reduces feelings of depression, helps you sleep better and helps maintain healthy bone, cartilage, muscles and more.

Stress also can take a serious toll on your physical health and quality of life. Everyone experiences stress at times. Negative events can cause stress: a crisis at work, an argument with your daughter, a bill that you don't know how you will pay. But happy events can stress you out, too: planning a wedding, packing for a vacation, sending your son off to college. Each person has a unique reaction to stress. Your blood pressure and body temperature might rise during stress, or you might lose or gain your appetite.

Stress is normal, but when you let stress persist for a long time, or get out of hand, it can hurt you. Excess stress can cause you to have headaches or chest pains, to grind your teeth, to abuse alcohol or drugs, and other unhealthy actions. Controlling stress is an important part of changing your life.

Now we come to an important question: If you do change your life, can you be absolutely sure you won't ever develop arthritis, diabetes, cancer, heart disease or other serious illnesses?

Unfortunately, the answer to that question is no. Nothing is guaranteed. You may know a person who smoked for many years, but lived a long life despite the habit that is proven to be unhealthy. You might know another person who seemed to diet and exercise sensibly, but still developed cancer, or arthritis or another serious health problem.

Every day it seems, we read about celebrities who develop serious health conditions or have to undergo surgery. Yet they seem so attractive, athletic and fit! Unfortunately, there is no guarantee that a seemingly fit, healthy-looking person won't develop an illness. But those people with a healthy weight, a physically fit body and a positive outlook often recover better from illness or surgery than a person who is overweight, out of shape and depressed.

What we do know is that unhealthy habits can increase your risk of disease, lower quality of life and pain. And it's proven that making even small, incremental changes to your eating, exercise and emotional habits can decrease your risk of those problems. Changing what you do can change the way you feel! It may take time, and it may take failing and starting over again. But you *can* change. You will feel better if you do change.

It's important to learn how to change in small, easy ways – like the ideas we offer in this book. That way, you don't have to feel that change is impossible and unattainable. You will see that you can take small steps to your long-term goal of losing weight, getting fit and improving your outlook on life.

Change – How Long Does It Take?

It's hard to say how long it takes to make positive changes in your lifestyle. It's even harder to determine how long it might take for you to see a difference that spurs you to continue your new, healthy habits.

Every person is different. For some people, making a significant change might take a few months, but for others, a year or more. It's easy to change for one day. But changing a habit and making it stick is a little harder!

Change Your Life shows you ways to keep track of your changes and be more accountable to yourself or others so those changes will last. Remember: Each small change you make and stick to will have a positive effect on your well-being. Before long, you will see the benefits of what you do for yourself every day, and you will be glad you've made these changes.

Changes can be difficult. If everyone liked eating broccoli as much as they liked eating pizza, it would be no problem convincing people to eat a healthy diet. You might eat high-fat foods because they taste yummy. So changing your diet to reduce overall fat intake – even if you know that this change will lead to a better weight – may feel like a loss to you. "I hate eating whole-wheat bread and vegetables. Yuck! Getting healthy isn't worth giving up the things I love to eat," you might say.

Don't look at changes as "giving up" or "sacrificing" things you like. Instead, look at some foods and activities as treats – such as a piece of chocolate cake, or time spent loafing on the couch watching a favorite old movie on TV. If your diet consists of mostly fatty, high-calorie foods, such as deep-fried chicken or onion rings, your diet would probably be pretty unhealthy. But if you try to eat a healthy diet most of the time, and enjoy your onion rings as a special snack once in a while, you'll still be able to achieve your goals.

How often can a "special treat" be eaten? That may vary from person to person. A treat might be enjoyed once a week for some people, or once a month for others. If you ate a piece of chocolate at the end of each workday as a "special treat," that might constitute an "everyday treat" rather than something special! One good trick is to find a substitute for your everyday sweets or snacks – perhaps a cup of fat-free hot chocolate or fat-free chocolate pudding (available in most supermarkets) for a low-calorie dose of sweetness. Once you get used to eating a food substitute that is lower in calories, you may find that you don't miss the higher-calorie choice!

It's important to make healthy choices your special rewards. For instance, exercise should not be a chore – it should be something that makes you feel good. Exercise may seem difficult at first, if you have not been doing any form of exercise. Later in this book, we'll show you ways to exercise that anyone can do, and ways to stay limber, so you lower you risk of pulling muscles or feeling soreness after you exercise. We'll also show you ways that you can overcome your own excuses for not exercising – for example, what to tell yourself when you say, "I'm too tired to exercise after work," or "I just don't like to exercise."

Everyone can exercise if they put their mind to do it. There is a form of exercise for every person – even for people who are in wheelchairs. The next time you say, "I can't do it," go watch a basketball game played by men and women in wheelchairs. Their determination will inspire you!

Setting Goals – Don't Reach for the Moon

One of the most important lessons in *Change Your Life* is learning to set goals that are attainable. If you aim for standards that only a professional athlete could achieve, what is the point of trying to change? Realize that you are only an ordinary human being who wants to improve. If you don't choose goals that are realistic, you will fail and you will wind up feeling worse than before. You'll feel like a failure, when all you really did was aim too high! Set your goals by understanding where you stand now – we'll show you how in Chapter Two.

Many people have an image of the person they could be if every aspect of their body and lifestyle was perfect – an image that is unrealistic. We all see pictures of beautiful fashion models or movie stars in magazines. They look impossibly thin and shapely. They seem to have

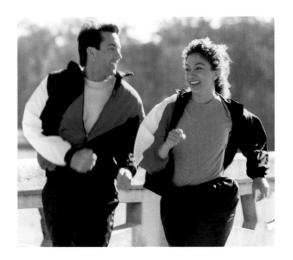

no skin flaws, no stomachs poking out underneath tight sweaters, no emotional problems or stress. Remember – these images are crafted carefully by advertising executives, publicists and photograph editors. They're not real! In addition, we all know people who seem "perfect" from our perspective. In reality, these people are not perfect – they have problems, fears, stresses and drawbacks, just like everyone else.

Resist the urge to compare yourself to others. You can only be the best person you can be. You can only attain the goals that you set for yourself.

We'll show you how to set goals that are realistic. What is an unrealistic goal? These are goals that involve a drastic, sudden switch from the lifestyle you have now to one you imagine. Let's say your diet consists mainly of items from the fast-food drive-through. On the way to work each morning, you scoot by the fast-food joint for a sausage biscuit and an order of fried hash browns. For lunch, you zip out for a hamburger and fries or a 12-inch pepperoni pizza (it's "personal size," you tell yourself). For dinner, you pick up a fried chicken and cheese submarine sandwich, more fries and a chocolate shake for dessert. Guess what? You're probably eating 3,000 calories to 4,000 calories a day. Unless you are a marathon runner, you're probably not burning most of these calories, and you need to lose some weight.

So you set a goal to lose weight. How will you accomplish your goal? If you are like many Americans, you might set an unrealistic, unattainable goal: "If I eat only plain, canned tuna and raw vegetables for the rest of the month, I'll lose at least 15 pounds!"

What would happen if you tried this radical "diet"? You might last about one or two days. Even though your new diet seems a lot healthier than the greasy fare you are used to consuming, your stomach would be in terrible pain from the drastic switch from low-fiber, fried foods to very high-fiber foods like raw vegetables. The deprivation of carbohydrates might make your digestive system revolt too. Mostly, you would feel deprived, bored by your new cuisine, and longing for the easy, tasty treats you love. "It would be so much easier just to swing through that drive-through window for a cheeseburger, instead of waiting until I get home to steam some fish…" Bad habits will return in force.

So you see, setting unrealistic goals means you may be setting yourself up for failure.

What is a realistic goal? A realistic goal is making gradual change. Examples of gradual change could include pledging to make a bowl of instant oatmeal at work for breakfast instead of eating your drive-through, greasy breakfast. Or, try this new breakfast every other day. After a few weeks, increase your new habit to every day. After that, you can build on that change. You might see if there are other, healthier choices on the fast-food restaurant's lunch menu. Most fast-food restaurants carry healthier items – have you looked? For lunch, try a grilled chicken sandwich instead of the fried variety. If you

can't part with fries all at once, try ordering the small size instead of the triple serving. Every other day, you might try to pair your sandwich with a salad instead of fries.

Soon, you will see that these types of goals – ones that involve small changes to your routine, or that require making healthier choices in the same situation – are easier to adjust to and easier to sustain than more aggressive, unrealistic goals. By making positive changes gradually, you will become used to doing things in a new way. Once a healthy choice becomes a healthy habit, you will see positive results in the way you look and feel.

NEVER SAY NEVER – LEARN TO COMPROMISE

Don't say you will never do something you like to do in order to try to attain your goals. For example, don't say, "I will never eat chocolate again, so I can be thin like the women I see in magazines." Making this kind of change can cause you to play against yourself – almost as if you are two people inside one person. One person wants to eat a healthier diet, but the other person likes eating chocolate. So the first person tells the second person to stop eating chocolate so she can achieve her goal. Except – you are one person!

You want to make positive changes, but you also like your treats. You are giving yourself an ultimatum – give up chocolate or you will suffer!

Get real. Who wants to be treated this way? Inevitably, you will side with the part of you that wants the chocolate, and you may seal this decision by overeating chocolate and giving up on your long-term, healthy goal.

Change by ultimate decree can be very unhealthy, because this is change that won't last. You may resent the change you are trying to make, and feel like you have to make unfair sacrifices in order to be healthier. You may get discouraged and give up on your larger goals.

Learn to compromise. If you love chocolate cake, you might try having a smaller slice of chocolate cake at first. Then, try choosing a reduced-fat, chocolate muffin at the supermarket bakery. These small compromises let you have your treats but keep your overall goals in motion. It's important to treat yourself once in a while. Later, we'll look at how you can find sensible ways to reward your great efforts.

One of the toughest challenges for most people is finding time in their schedule for doing the things that lead to good health. When you come home from work at the end of the day, you might like to grab the remote control, flip

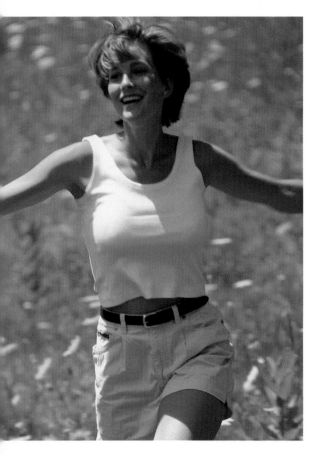

on your favorite TV game show and sit on the couch for a while. That makes you feel good! But, you realize that you are out of shape and need to get some exercise.

Looking over your schedule, you realize that after work is the only time you have to take a walk or ride a stationary bicycle. So you say to yourself, "If I have to exercise, I'll never be able to watch my game show again. I'll just give up my time vegging out in front of the TV." You might resent that change, even though it is a healthy change.

Why not strike a compromise? Perhaps you could push your stationary bicycle in front of the TV set, so you can pedal and watch TV at the same time. Or, you might alternate exercise and "veg time," going for a walk every other day. Or, you might tape your favorite show so you can watch it after you come back from your walk, at a time when there is nothing on that you like to watch.

The key to changing your life is finding things you can change, not things you cannot change, or will not change. It's important to look at your lifestyle and your routine objectively – we'll show you how!

Balance –
The Ultimate Goal for Everyone

Just as improving your diet and getting exercise are crucial to good health, it's also important to get the rest you need. For example, you must find ways to relax when you are experiencing stress in your life. As we said earlier, stress can cause many physical problems and make it difficult for you to achieve your goals.

Each person must learn to identify the things that cause stress, because what is stressful for

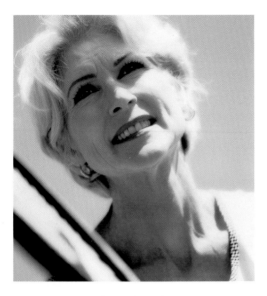

one person – packing for a business trip, going to visit in-laws, getting a new job – may not be stressful for another. So it's very important for you to find out what is causing your stress.

In Chapter Six, you will learn how to track the events that cause stress, and what type of reaction you detect in your body or mind when these events occur. You'll also find ways to relieve stress – positive, healthy therapies for stress. When you're experiencing stress, you might eat an entire carton of ice cream, or light up a cigarette even though you had wanted to quit once and for all. We'll suggest positive ways to relieve stress without hurting your health in other ways.

A healthy diet, regular exercise, stress relief. All of these elements blend together to form balance in your life. A balanced, healthier life is what you are trying to achieve, and what this book will try to help you attain. Not a perfect life, because perfection is not on the menu.

Again, don't compare yourself to someone else, or to a standard that is impossible to achieve. Find your own balance instead. Ask yourself what you can realistically do in your day-to-day life. Perhaps you can't exercise every single day. So start by exercising a few days a week, or by just being more active in your daily activities, like taking the stairs instead of the elevator. Breaking bigger goals into smaller ones will have a positive impact on your health. Just wait and see!

THE TIME TO CHANGE IS NOW

You might think, "You know, I would like to make changes in my life. I'm overweight, but I can't seem to start losing weight. The only exercise I get on most days is walking to the mailbox and back. Most days, I'm so stressed out after work that all I want to do is hit the couch with a tray of chili-covered nacho chips. I want to change. But I have no idea how to start, where to start or where to turn for help."

This is the place. This is the time. You can do it. You are worth the effort to make small changes that turn into big changes in how you feel.

Change Your Life will show you simple solutions – not drastic, unattainable ones – to lose some weight, get into an exercise routine and improve your outlook on life. We'll give you tips and activities to try, charts you can photocopy and fill out as you need them, advice from experts, and the inspiration you need to kickstart your efforts and keep them going.

Why wait one more minute to start making that change? *Let's get started!*

THE ROAD TO CHANGE:
WHERE are You NOW?

What's the first step in moving toward a healthier future?
Understanding where you stand today.

As you start your quest to make positive change, you need to know where you are now. To set goals, you must have a clear understanding of your starting point. In this chapter, we will look at ways to assess your state of health and fitness, and help you set goals that are attainable.

Experts on behavior modification – which is a fancy term for changing your unhealthy habits – use a scale to determine where someone is on the road to change. When people are going to stop a bad habit (say, overeating) or start a good one (say, exercise), they progress through fairly predictable stages.

Some of these stages may last a long time, even years. Some people move forward to the next stage, only to revert to the previous stage after some time has passed. Most people are at various stages throughout their life. You may,

for example, know someone who exercises regularly, but is a junk-food junkie. So this person has made better progress in the exercise department, but has some changes to make in terms of a nutritious diet. Understanding where you are on the road to change can give you insight into your own behavior. Knowing that change doesn't happen overnight can help you recognize the progress you've made, even if it isn't complete.

What Stage Are You In?

To begin, you need to identify what stage of health and fitness you are in now. Don't worry if you find that you are in the earliest stage. You have to start somewhere! Just accept where you stand and realize that once you make simple changes, you will progress to higher stages. Once you have made a commitment to yourself

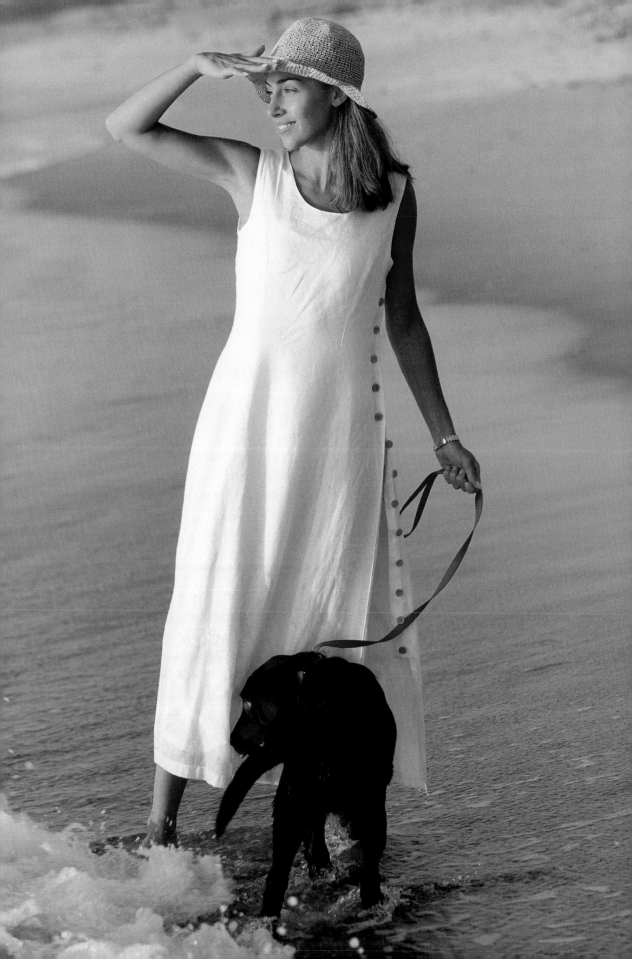

that you will make some changes, progressing will not be as difficult as you think it is now.

Here are the various stages on the road to change. Review the descriptions under each stage to determine where you fit. Once you are able to determine what stage you are in, you can then set goals to progress to higher stages. That's the overall goal – to reach a higher stage and a higher level of health and fitness.

Remember: Be honest with yourself. See what statements sound the most like your situation to determine your stage.

YOU ARE IN STAGE 1, IF

- You have no plans to start exercising. "Exercise just isn't for me."
- You don't intend to improve your diet. "I am not going to deprive myself of foods I love."
- You've gotten comfortable with your extra weight. "I'll just buy clothes one size bigger."
- You doubt your ability to do better. "I never stick with my diets (or exercise) anyway."
- You are defensive when others suggest that you exercise more or change your diet. "I am not that much overweight," or "I get enough exercise."
- You don't even notice your irritable mood when others do. "Grumpy? Who, me?"
- You don't believe there's anything that can be done for any of your health problems, such as arthritis, high blood pressure, chronic back pain or excess weight. "It can't be cured, so why bother?" Or, "This is my genetic make-up. I can't do anything about it. I just want to forget about it."

What You Should Know: You're in what experts call the "precontemplation stage." This term means that changing your behavior – improving your diet, increasing your level of

physical activity or reducing your stress – hasn't even crossed your mind.

Tip: Try reading some basic health education material, either at your doctor's office, your local library, bookstore or on the Internet. Talk with your doctor about the benefits you would get if you did make some small changes.

YOU ARE IN STAGE 2, IF

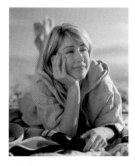

- You intend to eat better – eventually. "This year, I'm going to eat more vegetables."
- You intend to begin exercising – eventually. "I'm going to find a class in the spring."
- Your intentions are good, but you keep putting off healthy changes. "It's too cold to start walking now, but I'll do it when the weather warms up."
- You think but don't do. "Yeah, I've heard of a way to bake 'fried' chicken. Maybe I'll do it next time."
- You want to become a more involved patient. "I keep meaning to make a list of questions to take to my next doctor appointment."

What You Should Know: You are in what experts call the "contemplation stage." This term means you aren't taking any action, but you know you should take action. You may be a "chronic contemplator," someone who is more comfortable thinking about changes than actually making any moves.

Tip: Understand that your tendency is to think, not do. To overcome that, you'll need to push yourself. Just start slowly by setting small goals. Feel proud for even the small steps you take. Learn to "celebrate everyday victories." Later in the book, we'll explain this idea further.

YOU ARE IN STAGE 3, IF

- You have a plan to start exercising. "I have signed up for the water exercise class at the Y. It starts next month."
- You intend to eat better – soon, but not today. "I've subscribed to a healthy cooking magazine and will pick some recipes to try soon."
- You've got an idea for lightening your workload. "I'm writing up a proposal for hiring another employee at work."
- You've got a plan to reduce your stress. "I've already told them that I'm only going to join one committee for the upcoming fundraiser."

What You Should Know: You are in what experts call the "preparation stage." This means you have specific plans to put your health first. It might take a while, however, for you to get in gear.

Tip: Don't lose steam between making the plan and starting. Try to keep in mind the benefits you will reap once you get your routine under way.

YOU ARE IN STAGE 4, IF

- You have already made changes in your diet. "I've been cooking healthier versions of some of my favorite recipes."
- You have already begun to exercise. "I've been walking 20 minutes three times a week for a month now."
- You have begun counseling for your stress. "I'm seeing my pastor on a weekly basis now to talk about some of my personal struggles and work on reducing my stress."
- You have limited your obligations. "This year, I'm enjoying my son's Little League

games from the bleachers. Someone else is going to be coach."

What You Should Know: You are in what experts call the "action stage." This means you are doing it. Good for you! Be aware that, especially in the first six months of starting your new habits, setbacks can happen, temporarily knocking you off course. Don't worry. If that happens, just pick up where you left off.

Tip: Keep track of your daily successes to stay motivated. Keep a journal where you write down your thoughts, actions, challenges and accomplishments.

YOU ARE IN STAGE 5, IF

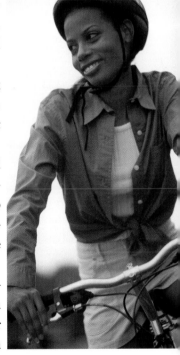

- You've been exercising for nearly a year. "I work out several times a week."
- You've been eating well for nearly a year. "I keep my diet in check."
- You have limited your extracurricular commitments to one at a time. "I volunteer for only one organization now."
- You have been taking 10 minutes a day to write in your journal for about a year now. "My journal helps me keep things in perspective."

What You Should Know: You are in what experts call the "maintenance stage." This means you have successfully started some new, healthy habits and maintained them for six months. Risk of relapse continues to decline as you continue your healthy ways.

Tip: Feel proud of your accomplishments – you've earned some self-praise. Work on your mindset by seeing these changes as permanent, rather than as habits you are "trying out." Think about how you will keep your good habits going even if life throws you a curve ball, such as if you start a new, high-stress project at work.

YOU ARE IN STAGE 6, IF

• You've been living a healthy lifestyle for more than five years. "I don't even have to think about it any more. I exercise regularly, eat well and keep my emotional health on an even keel. I don't see it as an option. These things are musts for me."

• You have a plan to put in action if problems occur in your life, so you won't backslide into old, bad habits of not exercising, eating junk food for dinner and letting stress take over. "I know that if things get bumpy, I can just buy pre-made healthy dishes at the supermarket for dinner. My husband knows I need to take time for a warm bath to relax my sore muscles and soothe my stress, so he can do the dishes. It's not a problem."

What You Should Know: You are in what experts call the "termination stage." This means you have maintained good habits for five years and have little chance of relapse. Your healthy habits are as automatic as brushing your teeth before bed.

Tip: What can we tell you? You're there. Keep up the good work and build on your success. Share your tips for making healthy habits a part of every day with other people!

Now that you have identified your stage, you know where to begin. On the next pages, you can take a brief quiz to find out more about your state of health, nutrition and fitness to further identify areas where you might need to make changes. You may find that in some areas, you are in a higher stage – such as exercise. You might exercise fairly regularly, but still struggle to eat a healthy, balanced diet, making your weight an ongoing problem. So concentrate on making changes to your diet while keeping up your exercise routine. When you have your dietary goals and your fitness activity at the same stage, then you can find ways to progress to a higher stage in both areas.

Don't try to do everything at once, or set goals that are too difficult for you to attain. That will only make it more difficult for you to maintain your change – the most important factor in this quest. We're looking for gradual changes here, not drastic changes that you will give up in a few weeks (or days).

In the following pages, you will get a few tips to keep in mind as you set your goals for change. You'll also find a variety of first-step goals to make the right changes for your health. Remember, if you find you need more specific guidance in any area, such as how you might get more calcium, you may wish to consult your doctor, a local nutritionist or dietitian.

Great Goals:
Make Your Resolutions a Reality

Those New Year's resolutions. So easy to make. So easy to break. Year after year, we envision an ideal version of ourselves. We make commitments. "I'm going to lose 30 pounds." "I'm going to give up fast food." But, honestly, did you ever

How Healthy Are You Living?

Here is a handy quiz to help you assess your current state of health. Remember, you probably aren't doing all or most of these things now, or why would you be reading this book? But this is a good way to see, in more concrete terms, what changes you need to make over the coming year.

Circle the number beside the answer that best describes your health habits. After each answer is a points value – keep track of your cumulative points to calculate your score and learn how healthy you are living.

Do you exercise?
3 yes, regularly
2 occasionally
1 rarely/never

Do you eat a healthy diet?
3 yes, mostly
2 about half and half
1 no

Do you drink plenty of water?
3 seven or eight 8-oz. glasses a day
2 four to six 8-oz. glasses a day
1 three or fewer 8-oz. glasses a day

Do you take a multivitamin supplement?
3 yes, regularly
2 occasionally
1 rarely/never

Do you feel you have a good support network of friends and/or family?
3 yes
2 so-so
1 no

Do you rest or relax periodically during the day?
3 yes, most days
2 occasionally
1 rarely/never

Do you take your prescribed medications regularly?
3 yes, most days
2 occasionally
1 rarely/never

Do you understand what your doctor tells you about your state of health?
3 yes
2 somewhat
1 no

Do you watch more than two hours of TV daily?
3 no
2 a little more
1 a lot more

Do you have trouble saying "no" to requests?
3 never
2 sometimes
1 always

Do you get regular checkups (blood pressure, mammograms, prostate screening, cholesterol, etc.)?
3 yes
2 for some things
1 no

continued on p.18

continued from p.17

Do you feel you get enough sleep?
3 yes, usually
2 occasionally
1 rarely/never

Do you have trouble falling asleep?
3 no, rarely or never
2 occasionally
1 yes, frequently

Do you get 1,000 milligrams to 1,200 milligrams of calcium daily?
3 yes, regularly
2 occasionally
1 no, rarely/never

Do you keep a journal?
3 yes, faithfully
2 occasionally
1 no

Are you in a loving relationship?
3 yes
2 in a relationship, but it could be more loving
1 no

Do you look forward to your day when you wake up in the morning?
3 yes, usually
2 sometimes
1 no, rarely/never

Do you know and use at least three nondrug ways to control pain?
3 yes
2 just one or two
1 no

Do you get angry or irritable daily?
3 no, rarely/never
2 sometimes
1 yes, regularly

Are you unusually tearful?
3 no
2 somewhat
1 yes

Do you read nutrition labels on food products to decide which to buy?
3 yes, usually
2 occasionally
1 no, rarely or never

Do you drink alcohol?
3 no, rarely/never
2 yes, in moderation
1 yes, frequently

Do you work more hours than you probably should?
3 rarely/never
2 sometimes
1 all the time

Scoring

Add your numbers to calculate your points score. If you scored above 55, you're doing great. Keep up the good work! If you scored 36-54, then you're doing pretty well but could use a few more healthy habits in your life. If you scored less than 35, now is the right time to pick five resolutions and get started on the road to changing your life.

really mean it? Whether you are picking up this book in January, May or October, make a pledge to get real. It's OK to vow to do better, but forget perfection and unattainable promises.

How can you keep your promises real? First, think about what you want to do or change. Then, get specific. State your goal in measurable terms. But don't stop there. Take that goal and make it even more real. Plan a first step toward your goal. Most of our goals are pretty lofty. We can get there eventually, but we forget that any destination is reached one step at a time. So decide how you will start. Once you've successfully completed the first step, plan your next one.

Consider the following goals. All of them are terrific – proven ways to improve your health, whether in changes to diet, fitness or other aspects of well-being. Which ones will you adopt? Check off five that suit you. Make these goals your own. You can amend the specifics so they work for you, or make a goal-setting contract form like the one on page 27. Some of these goals may be easy for you to achieve; you may be doing these things already. Others may be a struggle for you to build into your life. If you do struggle with some changes at first, don't give up entirely. Try to remember that some changes may be harder to incorporate into your routine, but all of these changes are attainable. Keep trying, and you will do it!

Think of each goal you set today as just that – a goal to achieve. Along the road to achieving any goal, you need to take small, first steps. You wouldn't run a marathon if you had never run a mile, would you? You would begin training for that marathon by running one mile, then two, then five, and so on, until you had slowly increased your endurance and ability to run the distance. You're not trying to run a marathon here – just to make some overall improvements to your lifestyle. But keep those long-term goals in mind as you "train" yourself through short-term goals and small changes.

Say these to yourself, or write in your journal:

I RESOLVE TO:

Drink more water.

Goal: Drink six to eight 8-ounce glasses of water daily.

First Step: Drink a full glass of water with each meal.

Eat less fat.

Goal: Get no more than 30 percent of my daily calories from fat.

First Step: Switch to skim milk, and low-fat or fat-free dairy products.

Eat more fiber.

Goal: Get 25 grams to 30 grams of fiber daily.

First Step: Add a high-fiber cereal to breakfast.

Get enough calcium.

Goal: Get 1,000 milligrams (mg) to 1,200 mg of calcium daily.

First Step: Take a calcium supplement to make up for diet shortage.

Fill in nutrition gaps in my diet.

Goal: Get at least the daily value of standard vitamins and minerals.

First Step: Get your doctor's advice on which vitamins you need and how much of each.

Eat more fruits and vegetables.

Goal: Get two to four servings of fruits and three to five of vegetables daily.

First Step: Have one piece of fresh fruit daily as a snack.

Begin an exercise program.

Goal: Do 20 minutes of exercise three times a week.

First Step: Walk for 10 minutes two times a week.

Exercise more consistently.

Goal: Do 20 minutes of exercise three times a week for a month.

First Step: Find a walking partner you can count on.

Boost my exercise program.

Goal: Take heart rate up to target range during exercise.

First Step: Identify your target range and learn how to measure heart rate.

Improve my flexibility or range of motion.

Goal: Do stretches daily.

First Step: Get directions from your doctor or physical therapist for five easy stretches to do twice a week.

Get enough sleep.

Goal: Get at least eight hours of sleep every night.

First Step: Tell friends and family you won't take calls past 9 p.m. – and stick to it.

Get enough rest.

Goal: Be off your feet for two hours each day.

First Step: Keep afternoons or early evenings unscheduled two days a week to allow for "chill" time.

Reduce my level of stress.

Goal: Reduce number of things on your to-do list.

First Step: Identify two to-do items each week that you can delegate to someone else or not do at all. It might not make a difference if some things don't get done!

Wow! Now you have some clear, concrete goals for making positive changes in your life, and some basic first steps to get you started. You will find that once you make small changes, these new habits will become routine. Your body will tell you when you are not doing what is best for it.

Once you begin getting more activity, exercise will become a little easier. You will feel less energy if you don't get your exercise. Once you begin eating a more healthful diet, eating nutritiously won't seem so strange. You may even find that your body reacts negatively to eating a large, fat-laden meal. You might feel stuffed and sluggish. In turn, that feeling will reinforce your body's desire to have more wholesome, nutritious fare. In Chapter Four, we'll provide some recipes and resources for you to create easy, wholesome, nutritious meals.

Later in this chapter, you'll get some guidance in how to set a game plan for yourself as you begin the road to change. You will make a contract with yourself, setting a simple, attainable goal and making a pledge to keep to that goal. You can keep this contract just with yourself, or have a friend, family neighbor or your doctor sign it also. You choose how to do this – it may help you to have someone else motivate you, or it may seem like too much pressure at first.

You also will want to track the changes you make by keeping a journal or record of what

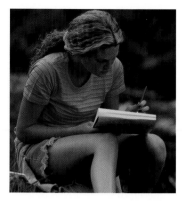

you eat, how you exercise and how you feel on a daily basis. This is not the type of journal you kept in junior high – it's a way to monitor what you are doing, and to identify areas where you may be struggling. Let's talk about how you can do this.

Keep It Up by Keeping Tabs

Studies have shown that people who record, or write down in some way, their attempts to improve their health do better in the long run. You can use a journal to set goals, record what you eat and how much, or keep a log of your exercise – what you did, for how long and how you felt before and after. Likewise, putting your goals in writing increases the odds that you'll stick with the plans you have for putting yourself first.

OK, you might say, "I just don't have time to keep a journal. I'm not a writer. I'm not good at keeping track of things in general – why would I keep up with writing all this stuff down in a journal? I won't remember to do it."

First, you don't have to write in this journal every single day, although it will help your efforts immensely if you do. Some days, it won't be convenient for you to sit down and write. That's OK. Do it as often as you can.

To make journaling easier, don't think that you have to fill up an entire page, or even write in paragraphs. You can make a list, or jot a few things down. Make keeping your journal an easy task, not a chore, so you can do it every day. You can do as little as recording what you ate and if you exercised or not.

Decide what things are most important for you to keep track of. Then buy a journal, photocopy the sample from this book or design your own log and goal sheet. It's up to you.

Think of how and when you will use your journal. Some people like to keep their journal close at hand; others post it where it can't be missed – on the refrigerator, the bathroom mirror or beside their bed so they see it last thing at night or first thing in the morning. What you write is up to you. Don't worry about spelling and grammar. No one but you will see what you write!

If you like, indulge in a pretty or portable blank book so journaling seems like something special. You can purchase these journals at most stores that sell stationery or paper products. The Arthritis Foundation publishes a journal called *Toward Healthy Living: A Wellness*

6 Tips for Success

- Set goals. Be specific. Be realistic.
- Break each goal into doable steps. Take them one at a time.
- Expect setbacks. Just pick up where you left off.
- Get a buddy to work with you.
- Keep a journal or a log of your progress.
- Believe in yourself. You have what it takes to accomplish your goals!

Journal, with charts to track your mood and physical well-being, as well as inspirational quotes to keep you going. See the resources section at the end of this book to find out more about helpful Arthritis Foundation products and services like this one.

Whatever you do, don't lose track of your daily successes. These successes tell you where you're going and why. It's important for you to keep an eye on your progress, so you will realize where you are moving forward in your changes and where you may need reinforcement. If you write down your actions on a regular basis, you will be more accountable to yourself. And, you will clearly see the changes you are making and the positive impact they are having on your life.

We suggest that you keep one diary for tracking all three areas of change we are discussing in this book:

- Diet
- Exercise
- Outlook

However, if you are just focusing on one or two areas of change, and not all three, it's OK just to keep a diary with this information. It's up to you. You may wish to monitor diet and exercise on a daily basis, and only note events related to your stress or personal outlook when they occur. You are the best judge of your personal needs when it comes to change.

WHAT YOU NEED TO KEEP TABS ON

What sort of things should you write in your journal? You may wish to record a variety of different daily activities or feelings. Some people enjoy writing in a journal and making note of the challenges they face in accomplishing their goals. You may not be that ambitious. But you should at least write down the following things on a daily basis if possible:

- Daily food and beverage intake, including portion sizes, such as "three handfuls of mixed nuts from the bowl at the party, plus one light beer"
- Daily exercise, including time and distance, and even incidental exercise, like "taking the stairs instead of the elevator at work"
- Daily or periodic episodes of stress, or when you find that you experience a change in your stress levels, such as "reacted more calmly to a damaged blouse at dry cleaner than I usually do"
- Personal challenges and triumphs, such as "had to discuss my raise with my boss today – went to the snack machine for some potato chips afterward"

It's OK to record your feelings in your journal, including how you feel about your efforts to make changes, and what areas you find difficult to change.

Remember – this is *your* Changes Journal. Don't share it with anyone if you don't want to. It is meant to help you keep track of how you are doing, but you don't need to answer to anyone about your progress, except yourself and possibly, your doctor.

Your Changes Journal

At the end of this book, you'll find some sample journal pages that you can photocopy and use for your own needs. As we said earlier, you can buy a blank journal or a spiral-bound weekly calendar book and create your own Changes Journal.

Start your journal by reviewing the basic goals we discussed earlier in this chapter. Think about which goals are most important for you. Do you need to eat more fruits and vegetables, or exercise, or get enough rest? And don't forget: You may not be able to focus on all these goals in the beginning, or incorporate all the recommended "first steps" all at once. Choose the ones that are most important and applicable to your situation.

Then, set some personal goals for the next month. These might be:

My Goals for January:

- Take my vitamin supplement each morning.
- No snacking after dinner or after 8 p.m. each night.
- Do my range-of-motion stretches every morning.
- Try the yoga video I bought last year but never unwrapped.

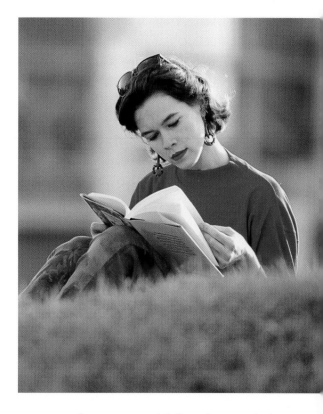

Then, you will set up areas to record the three categories of change for each day of the week. For example, under Monday, January 1, you would set up three columns for diet, exercise and outlook. You may also add sections for challenges and triumphs. You can note these events or feelings as they occur.

Recording challenging or inspiring events and how you may have reacted to them – such as responding to losing a big sale at work by eating a large bag of cookies or by skipping your scheduled workout – can be helpful in your long-term efforts to change.

You can identify how you react negatively – or even positively – to various types of events in your life. Let's say you noted in your Changes Journal that you reacted to losing a sale one week by eating a bag of cookies. But the next time you experienced a stressful event at work,

you notice that you reacted differently. Instead of wolfing down a bag of cookies, you worked out your feelings by doing your scheduled routine on the treadmill. That's a triumph! You not only chose to work through your anxiety in a positive, healthy way, but you also learned a valuable lesson about how to deal with stress in your life.

Going back and reviewing how you reacted to various events will help you identify patterns in your behavior. These may be negative patterns that you wish to change, or positive patterns that you wish to continue.

Try to review your Changes Journal once a week to identify areas of progress and things you need to adjust. At the end of each week (whatever day you choose to mark the end of your week), sit down and go over the last seven days of journal entries. Take note of any problems you had – such as dealing with what to order on lunches out with work colleagues. Think about how you might handle these challenges more positively in the coming week. You might consider, for example, suggesting a restaurant that has healthier choices on the menu. Or rounding up your coworkers for a brown bag picnic outside one day, and bring yourself a healthy meal prepared at home.

HOW TO RECORD ITEMS
IN YOUR CHANGES JOURNAL

In the Diet section of your journal entries, note all the foods you eat each day, including portion size. You will need to learn to measure the portions of food you eat at first, until you get a clear idea of the "sensible portion size" of any particular food. You may consider investing in the following measurement tools if you don't have them now. These items should be available at most discount stores or cooking supply stores:

- a food scale
- a set of measuring spoons
- a liquid/dry measuring cup

These items will help you measure the amount of the foods you eat each day. Start by measuring one cup of dry cereal and one cup of skim milk. You may be surprised to learn that the amount of cereal you used to consider "one serving" was actually closer to two! In Chapter Four, we'll look at some easy ways to determine healthy portion sizes of various foods.

In the Exercise section, you should note the type of exercise you do each day, or if you do no exercise at all. You should note the duration of exercise, such as the time spent doing the exercise, as well as the distance you ran, walked, biked or swam, for example. Make sure you include inci-

> *"I've been cooking healthier versions of my favorite recipes."*

dental exercise you do during the day. If you walked up the stairs at work instead of taking the elevator, write it down. If you walked three blocks to the bank during your lunch break, write it down. Every bit of exercise counts – even if it seems like the normal things you do in your day. All those little bits of activity can add up.

It's helpful to track exercise by measuring what you do. This method keeps your efforts more organized and regular. You can time your exercise by using a timer on a treadmill or by tracking your walk with your watch. You could also measure the distance you exercise, such as walking four times around a quarter-mile track or by measuring your walking route using your car odometer.

In the Outlook section of your journal, you can record the events that cause you stress or emotional reactions to various events. These events are called stressors. Stressors can be both negative and positive. If a customer at work yells at you and calls you incompetent, this is a stressor. If you just got engaged and are now planning when and where to get married, this is a stressor too. Note these stressors as they occur, and write down how you reacted to them – for example, if you ran to the freezer to eat ice cream afterward, or if you took a hot bath instead.

If your goals include weight loss, it's a good idea to record your weight fluctuations in your journal. We recommend that you don't weigh yourself every day, however. Weight fluctuates for many people, due to various factors that may be beyond your control. If you check your weight every day, you may become too obsessed with small ups and downs and become discouraged about your progress.

We recommend weighing yourself weekly and recording this weight in your journal. As far as weighing yourself, follow these general guidelines:

- Pick one time each week to weigh yourself and stick to this time as often as possible.
- Wear the same clothing or type of clothing each time you weigh. Don't wear shoes.
- Use the same scale each time you weigh. Buy a new, calibrated scale if you think your current scale is too old or inaccurate.
- Write down your weight in your journal immediately after weighing. Then, don't look at it again until the next week!

You've made a great start – you have some goals for changing aspects of your life, a journal to record your diet, exercise and outlook for each day, and you have some first steps toward those goals. What you can do to really get started and focused on your goals is set up a "contract" with yourself, stating the specific goals you wish to accomplish and the specific steps you will try to take to get there.

Strategies for Journaling and Contracting

Change Your Life invites you to assume responsibility for making changes in your life. You can't change everything in your life, only the aspects you can control. For instance, you can control what you eat most of the time. You can't control what dishes are being served at your office holiday party but you can control what you actually put in your mouth at that party. The key is to make healthy choices so you stay in control.

There will always be things in your life that you cannot control. An account may fall through at work. Your mother may come down with a chronic illness and require long-term care. Snowy weather may make it impossible for you to take your daily walk in the neighborhood. You may find yourself at an all-day meeting where your client is serving pizza and garlic bread for lunch.

What you can control is how you react to things that are beyond your control. You can learn from past situations and mistakes. You can plan ahead when possible for challenges that may occur.

Instead of falling apart over an account falling through, you might sit down with someone else, such as a coworker or a friend, to find solutions to the problem.

Instead of letting your stress get out of control because of the account falling through or your mother's illness, you might find a way to release your stress, such as taking a warm bath.

Instead of using the snowstorm as an excuse to stay inside eating roasted marshmallows instead of exercising, you might pop in an exercise videotape and cook some vegetable pasta soup.

Instead of just eating three slices of pizza and a hunk of garlic bread at the all-day meeting, you could tell yourself to bring a salad or some healthy snacks to the meeting, and just have one slice of the pizza.

You won't be able to do the right thing all the time. As we said earlier, you will have to focus on learning from your challenges so you can react differently next time something occurs. Techniques discussed earlier in this chapter, such as goal-setting and contracting, can be very useful in helping you identify problems and solutions. They can help you stay on track. You can make a contract with yourself to accomplish small steps in achieving your larger goals.

MAKING A CONTRACT

Chart your course of action by using the sample contract provided on the next page. Describe each goal in realistic, very specific terms. Think of what you would like to do, and determine which of those things you can accomplish in the next several weeks or months. Don't get grandiose visions of yourself running marathons if you don't even run to the mailbox now. If you choose a goal that is too big or that will take too long, you may become discouraged and give up before you reach it.

In this contract, you'll need to break down your goal into smaller steps or tasks. These steps make reaching your goal more manageable. These steps also will give you a sense of accomplishment along the way so you can track your progress. For example, if your goal is to get in better physical shape, you might include these steps:

1. Make an appointment with your doctor or a physical therapist to discuss the best exercise options for you.
2. Find out about exercise classes and programs in your area.
3. Choose one and get started.

A contract is a way of making your goal more formal, and clearly identifying the steps you plan to take to reach it. Here are the steps:

1. What, specifically, you will do.
2. How much you will do.
3. When you will do it.
4. How often you will do it.

By creating this contract, you'll give yourself more of an obligation to fulfill your goal. Again, make this contract realistic. Staying real means contracting to do something three or four times a week, but not every day. Remind yourself that things come up that you cannot control.

Let's say you contract to walk every day after work. But your neighbor's father dies, and you and your family have to pay a sympathy call after work. You find that on this day, it's more important for you to sit with your neighbor for a while, talking with her and sharing a cup of coffee. So you don't have time to take your walk. You feel as if you have broken your contract and messed up one of your goals.

But if you set a more realistic contract of walking four times a week, you can make adjustments to stay with your goal despite what comes up. You have to go to visit your neighbor tonight, but tomorrow night you can walk.

How can you decide if your goal is realistic for you? Think about yourself now and what changes you hope to make. How sure are you that you can really achieve your goal? For example, on a scale of zero (completely unsure) to 10 (completely confident), you should have a confidence level of seven or greater that you can make these changes and meet the terms of your contract with yourself.

To stay motivated, get someone else, like a family member or close friend, to sign the contract too. Be sure you ask someone who is supportive of your quest to change. You don't need a taskmaster, but a cheerleader. If your "witness" is someone you live with or see often, they will probably see how your progress is going. They will be able to see if you are struggling to take your first steps, or if you are giving up, and hopefully, they will encourage you to keep going.

Try this sample contract and see how it works for you. We think this is a good strategy for identifying specific goals and how you will begin to achieve them.

Sample Contract

Name:_____

Goal:_____

Date Started:_____

Times To Check Progress: _____

This Week I Will:_____

What:_____

How Much: _____

When: _____

How Many Times:_____

Example:

Name: *Cindy Jones*_____

Goal: *To increase my activity level through regular walks.*_____

Date Started: *January 17*_____

Times To Check Progress: *The 17th day of each month for six months*

This Week I Will: *Walk around the neighborhood for 15 minutes after work three nights.*

What: *Walk*_____

How Much: *For 15 minutes*_____

When: *After work*_____

How Many Times/Days: *Three nights a week*_____

How Certain Are You?:_____

Scale: 0 (Completely Unsure) to 10 (Completely Confident)

Signature:_____

Witness (if needed):_____

Date:_____

Where To Go From Here

Great start! You have assessed where you stand now in your health, fitness and stress control ability. You have identified what "stage" you are in, so you know where you hope to go from here. You have learned a number of overall goals, and smart first steps to take in achieving these goals. You have a sample contract to sign with yourself (and with a friend or loved one as a witness, if you choose), and you have learned the benefits of keeping a journal or some other written record of your efforts and progress.

So, why not get started? There is no time better than now to set new goals and get to work on making them reality. The sooner you start your quest to change your life, the sooner you will see results in the way you look, feel and react to everything around you. Your journal entries will serve to encourage you as you go along.

REWARDING YOURSELF

As you begin, keep one important thing in mind: Celebrate everyday victories. That is one of the things this book will insist that you do. You like to celebrate – who doesn't? – and there's no better way to reinforce your success.

The challenge is to learn how to identify when you have an "everyday victory" and find positive, healthy ways to celebrate those triumphs. An example of an everyday victory might be achieving your exercise goal one week without any snags. Or it might be going to the local hamburger joint with friends and ordering a green salad with your hamburger instead of the chili cheese fries you used to think you couldn't live without. An everyday victory might be when you react to your mother-in-law's weekly phone call by staying calm instead of letting her nagging and criticisms get to you.

When these great things happen, note them in your journal. Think about this accomplishment: What steps did you take that were different that allowed you to achieve something that formerly seemed impossible? What tactics did you take to make a goal a reality? Once you have identified a strategy that worked for you – such as playing some upbeat background music during your mother-in-law's phone call to distract you a bit – resolve to try this again.

Now – how do you celebrate your victory? Don't celebrate the fact that you made a healthy

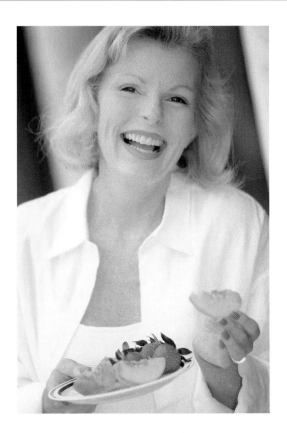

decision by doing something unhealthy. So you ordered the green salad instead of chili cheese fries. Don't order a hot fudge sundae for dessert as a reward. Do something healthy for yourself instead. Take a hot bubble bath. Watch one of your favorite old movies on video. Take some time on the weekend to hit golf balls at the driving range. Buy yourself a fun magazine that doesn't have to do with work.

Make time to celebrate your victories – this goal is as important as your other goals. Remember to congratulate yourself along the way for sticking to your efforts. Encourage yourself and be your own cheerleader, critic and coach all in one. If you are not resolved to change, nobody can make you change and you will not change. But if you find ways to congratulate, correct and motivate yourself, you will change!

CELEBRATE Your Success SMARTLY... and Stay MOTIVATED

Positive first steps are a great way to start. But you will only achieve success through sustained change. Staying motivated with the following tips will help you reach your goal.

In the previous chapter, we showed you how to assess what stage of action you are in now, in terms of your health, fitness and well-being. If you are in Stages 5 or 6, it's very likely that you don't need to learn ways to create a healthy diet or how to exercise – you're already doing these great things for yourself.

But most of us are in the earlier stages. We may know that we need to make changes to improve our health, and we may or may not know what changes will really help. What we need are simple strategies for getting started, and lessons in how to stay motivated once we get going. Nothing feels worse than starting a positive routine and then giving it up to go back to our negative habits. We feel like failures when we do that, but it's important that you put the "failure" concept out of your mind for good.

Everyone makes mistakes or has a lapse in their efforts to change. Everyone finds themselves in a situation – a dinner with important clients at a restaurant, for example – where it's difficult to find something healthy to eat. From time to time, you may find yourself eating a heavy meal or skipping your scheduled exercise routine for one reason or another. The important thing is to view those events as a pause in your quest, not a break.

Don't give up. Just get back to your routine as soon as you can. Don't beat yourself up about it, just put it behind you. Keep looking forward, and learn to celebrate when you do something good for yourself.

Make Time for a Healthier You

As you begin to make some simple changes to your lifestyle, you may encounter some all-too-

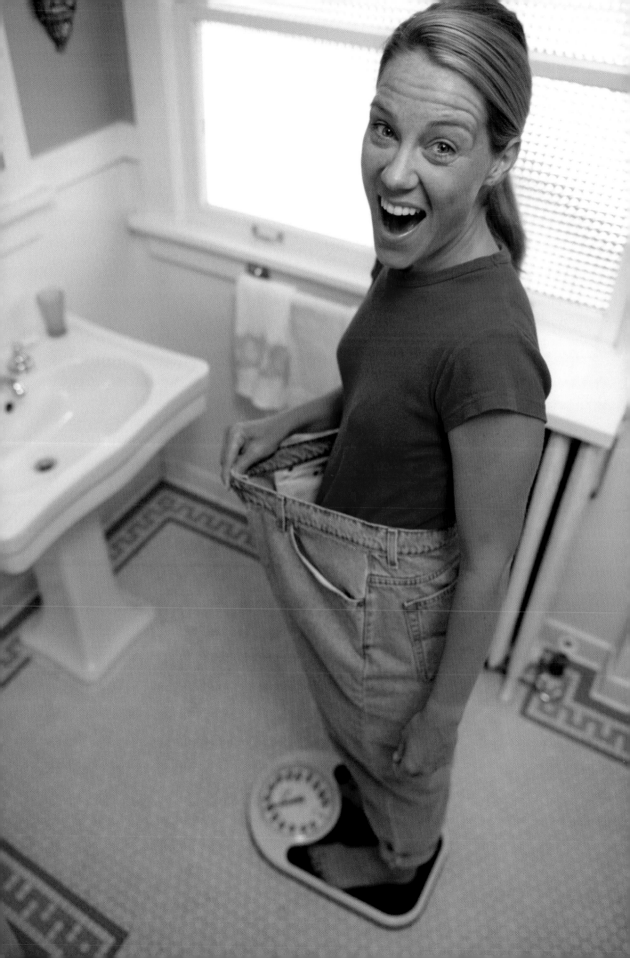

familiar roadblocks. These are the same problems that have derailed your diet or fitness efforts in the past.

Perhaps you find it too time-consuming to create healthy meals, when it's so much easier to drive through the fast-food restaurant on the way home, or pop a frozen pizza in the oven. Maybe you don't feel that you have the time to exercise when you also have a full-time job, two kids and a house to clean. And who has time to spend a half-hour soaking in a stress-relieving, warm bubble bath when the kids need to be put to bed and your spouse wants to go over the household finances...again?

One problem that many people encounter again and again 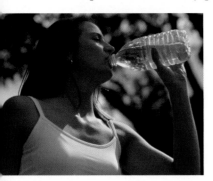 is the perception of a lack of time. This is one of the most common excuses (see Chapter Five) that people offer for not exercising at all. It's true – we all lead busy, frantic lives. We feel that we don't have time to do the things we have to do, the things that other people depend on us to do, much less the things we would like to do. But isn't it important for you to be healthy?

Other people in your life may or may not understand when you say, "I can't do that right now. I have to take a walk." With your jam-packed schedule, it may be very difficult for you to find time to work in healthy food, physical activity or much-needed "down time." Here, we offer some very simple strategies for doing just that – without adding much or any time to your already congested schedule. You probably can't

adopt all of these strategies, but you will find that some of them fit into your routine easily. Any of them will help you add health and balance to a life that needs those additions!

MAKE EVERY DAY A HEALTHY DAY

Here are plenty of ways to help you use each waking hour to the fullest. Try the following strategies to help you squeeze in more exercise, healthier food and emotional solace into your days and nights:

EARLY MORNING (6 A.M. – 9 A.M.)

- Take time to eat a healthy breakfast. Try oatmeal with a fruit topping, raisin toast and peanut butter or a fruit smoothie.
- Go for a quick walk around the neighborhood or do some light stretches.
- Meditate for 10 to 20 minutes; focus your mind on positive thoughts; set goals for the day or read an inspirational verse.

MID-MORNING (9 A.M. – 12 P.M.)

- Eat a healthy mid-morning snack. Grab a piece of fruit, a small bag of pretzels or a cup of yogurt.
- Monitor your posture. Sit up straight in your car, at your desk or while relaxing in front of the television.
- Focus on breathing correctly – your belly should move the most, not your chest.

EARLY AFTERNOON (12 P.M. – 3 P.M.)

- Opt for frozen meals for lunch that offer healthy options (low-fat, low sodium).
- Walk to lunch and enjoy the scenery or use this time to do your favorite workout video.
- Eat your lunch at a local park – no phones, no lists, no stress.

MID-AFTERNOON (3 P.M. – 5 P.M.)

- Squash your sweet tooth. Some experts say brushing your teeth can eliminate a sugar craving.
- Take a 10-minute walk break.
- Look both ways before you type – stretch your neck while you're seated at your desk.

EARLY EVENING (5 P.M. – 7 P.M.)

- Say no to second helpings and replace dessert with a cup of decaffeinated, flavored tea.
- Stretch at red lights – neck rotations, shoulder shrugs or wrist twists are helpful.
- Ask a neighbor or friend you haven't seen in a while to come over and take a walk with you instead of talking on the phone.

EVENING (8 P.M. – 10 P.M.)

- Enjoy a healthy evening snack if you're hungry. Try not to eat too close to bedtime.
- Tidy up your house a bit before bedtime. Vacuum one room, load the dishwasher or dust. Any type of movement keeps your body limber.
- Enjoy your favorite sitcom. Laughter is good medicine.
- Take a warm bath.

LATE EVENING (10 P.M. – 12 A.M.)

- Forgo the urge to snack so close to bedtime. If you must, try fruit or a high-fiber cereal.
- Write in a journal, catch up on some letter/postcard writing or get ready for the next day to reduce morning stress.
- Unplug your phone, curl up with a good book.

NIGHT OWLS (12 A.M. – 6 A.M.)

- Try a cup of warm milk or hot, decaffeinated tea if you wake up in the middle of the night.
- Gently tighten and release your muscles starting with your face and moving down to your toes.
- Count sheep, count backwards from 1,000 or picture yourself on a beach to induce sleep.

Overall, try to remember to take small steps. Incorporate just one change each week if that is all you can do. After eight weeks, you would have made eight healthy changes. That's incredible! You will see a tremendous impact on your well-being "bottom line" from just a few small changes like the ones suggested above.

In Chapter Four, we'll show you some easy ways to incorporate healthy food into your regular diet without completely "gutting" your normal eating plan all at once. In Chapter Five, we'll look at some simple suggestions for getting more physical activity and flexibility. In Chapter Six, we'll examine some stress-reduction and fatigue-fighting strategies that will help you have more energy to live each day.

SMALL CHANGE, BIG DIFFERENCE

Can a small change, such as substituting a healthy snack for a highly caloric one, really make a difference? It can – if you keep it up. It's really just basic math! Over time, a small subtraction adds up to a big deficit.

Let's say you made one small change – such as replacing your usual nighttime snack of a chocolate-covered ice-cream bar (300 calories) with a whole-grain, fruit-filled cereal bar (140 calories). What impact would you see on how much "snack time" adds to your total caloric intake for the week?

Before Change	After Change
One Week:	
2,100 calories	980 calories
Two Weeks:	
4,200 calories	1,960 calories

Before Change	After Change
Three Weeks:	
6,300 calories	2,940 calories
Four Weeks:	
8,400 calories	3,920 calories

In one month, you would have saved 4,480 calories just by making one small change from one sweet treat to another sweet treat. While you may feel that fruit-filled cereal bars aren't as tasty as chocolate-covered ice-cream bars, couldn't you think of a lot of other ways to spend more than 4,000 calories? Or if you saved those calories and didn't consume them in that month, don't you think you would see an impact? You would – even if your goal was just to maintain your current weight.

It takes 2,300 calories per day for a 165-pound, 45-year-old woman to maintain her current weight. That's 16,100 calories per week. If she spends 2,100 calories of that 16,100 total on that one dessert, she is consuming about 15 percent of her weekly calories on one snack. She could spend less than half of those calories on her snack, and save the rest for a special occasion dinner, a brunch out with her friends on the weekend, or not spending the calories at all and seeing an impact on her "bottom line" – her weight.

To make one small change such as this one – to substitute a high-calorie snack for a more sensible, nutritious one – is in itself a small victory. Once you have made a change and stuck to it for a month, you may think it's time to celebrate. Why? Because before you made this change, you may have thought that you could never change. You could never enjoy eating something healthy in place of something more "sinful." But then you discovered that this change was possible, and you made this change because you wanted to see a positive result that would last.

So, it's time to celebrate. How should you mark this victory? If you said you should celebrate by eating the ice-cream bar, keep reading and see why you may want to find something else.

Celebrate Everyday Victories

At the end of the last chapter, we brought up the idea of celebrating everyday victories. What is an everyday victory? What does it take to make you feel victorious?

You probably remember the thrill of beating your tennis opponent or whispering "check mate" to an old friend. The sweet smell of victory comes anytime you defeat an opponent or overcome an obstacle. If you have a health problem or a chronic illness such as arthritis, fibromyalgia, diabetes or others, it's quite clear who – or should we say what – the opponent is. Your obstacles may be anything from pain and fatigue to weight gain and mood swings.

But how do you know if you've been victorious against your inner and outer foes? For some, victory means being able to walk a marathon, for others it's being able to walk a mile and for some it's making it to the mailbox. We think victory is yours alone to define.

With victory should come reward. If losing 20 pounds is your goal, don't wait until you lose all

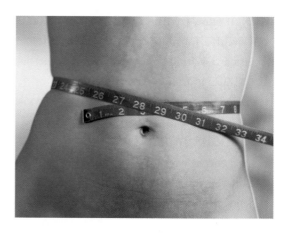

20. Go ahead and celebrate – pound by pound, step by step. Did you take the stairs instead of the elevator today? Reward yourself with a little self-praise or even a new self-help book.

Your goals are unique, so your rewards should be too. But why reward yourself for "baby steps" toward your ultimate goal? It's all about what you should be doing – motivating yourself to keep doing it. Otherwise you may find yourself stuck in a rut, retreating to old, bad habits.

But don't let rewards turn into obstacles and setbacks, either. A big slice of chocolate cake is obviously not the best reward for sticking to your no-sweets goal.

Making improvements in the role exercise, nutrition and emotional well-being play in your life can make a huge difference in how you feel. Taking on this challenge may seem daunting. On the way to achieving your health goals there are temptations (ice cream cake, holiday goodies from a neighbor, lounging on the couch) and obstacles (fatigue, hectic schedules, work assignments, health problems), but sometimes you beat them. When you do, it's time to celebrate.

As we said in Chapter Two, it's important to find positive ways to celebrate your success. Celebratory acts should reinforce the change you are making in your life, not undermine it. If you find that you have lost five pounds in your quest to change your eating habits and lose excess weight, would you celebrate by eating an entire chocolate cake in one sitting? You might wind up gaining back some of the weight you just lost, but more importantly, you have created an association between unhealthy habits and reward.

Instead of taking a step backward when you have reached a victory point, perhaps you can think of other ways to celebrate.

FINDING ALTERNATIVE WAYS TO CELEBRATE

It's helpful to make a list of things that you enjoy doing that don't involve food. Food is an integral part of celebration, but when celebrating with food or alcoholic beverages, many people have a tendency to overindulge on these treats. You will, at times, celebrate with food, but it may be helpful to learn other ways to mark your victory.

Sit down with a clean piece of paper or journal page and a pen. Think for a few minutes about things you like to buy yourself (these items can be small

Reward Yourself Right!

Here are a few ideas for celebrating everyday victories in a positive, reaffirming way.

VICTORY: Lost five pounds in five weeks.
CELEBRATION: Organize a berry- or apple-picking outing with your family.

VICTORY: Exercised according to the monthly goals you set.
CELEBRATION: Have your spouse watch your kids while you go to the mall for an hour, or soak in a warm bubble bath with a celebrity gossip magazine.

VICTORY: Made it through your office holiday party without eating any fried foods, cheese balls or cream pastries. Kept to your healthy eating plan all night long while still enjoying yourself.
CELEBRATION: Spend a weekend afternoon hitting golf balls at the driving range with your son and daughter.

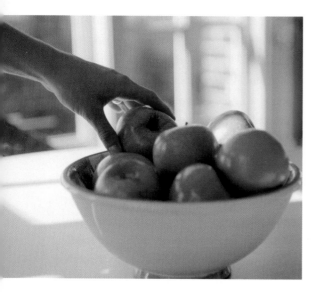

Moderation is the key to celebrating with food and alcohol. You've probably heard this term before, and it is hard to achieve for most people. But enjoying everything in moderation is essential if you are to stay in control of your weight, stress and other wellness factors.

Perhaps you would like to celebrate by savoring a glass of wine before dinner, after a long week of working hard to keep everything under control. That's OK – but don't turn one glass of wine into four glasses, followed by frantic munching of cheese crackers. ("I needed something in my stomach to counteract all the wine!")

Or you might like to splurge on a slice of apple pie after dinner. If so, take a look at the "serving size" indication on a packaged pie at the grocery store. Often, the recommended serving size will be 1/8 or even 1/12 of a whole pie – not a quarter of the pie. In Chapter Four, we'll look at the concept of serving sizes to help you understand what moderation means with various foods. You may wish to discuss this concept with your doctor, or with a registered dietitian or nutritionist, professionals who can help you conceive a personalized eating plan, and can work with you to tackle problems you may have with your diet.

and inexpensive) or like to do to celebrate. Perhaps it is a new CD by your favorite band; playing a computer golf game for an hour, uninterrupted; buying a bottle of a new nail polish; cruising the flea market on a Saturday morning. Whatever you enjoy that doesn't involve or revolve around eating or drinking alcohol.

Then make a list of the top ten things (or activities) and consult this list each time you have a victory. If you can substitute one of the items on this list for a food-oriented activity (such as a trip to the ice-cream parlor), you have achieved another victory of sorts.

It's OK if you enjoy celebrating with food. Consider celebrating by eating a new, exotic fruit bought from the farmer's market or the international section of your local supermarket. If you would rather celebrate with sweets, high-calorie foods like cheese, or beer, you can find a way to enjoy these treats without going overboard.

There is nothing wrong with treating yourself once in a while, particularly when you have something to celebrate. The key is to find a balance between doing what you like and doing what is right for your body.

When it comes to alcohol, each person is different. If you take certain medications on a regular basis, or if you have a health condition such as diabetes or gout (a disease related to arthritis), it may be unhealthy for you to drink any alcohol at all. There have been some studies that show a possible link between moderate consumption of red wine and a lowered risk of heart disease, but you should not misinterpret this finding to mean that the more red wine you drink, the lower your risk of disease.

If you are confused about how much alcohol is appropriate for you to drink, and how often,

Healthy Ways To Celebrate

Brainstorm some healthy ideas for celebrating your victories. Pull this list out when you need to perk yourself up or celebrate something to be proud of!

FIVE THINGS I LIKE TO DO
THAT DON'T INVOLVE FOOD
Samples: Listening to my favorite CD. Taking a countryside drive with the sunroof open. Hitting golf balls at the driving range. Reading to my grandchildren.

1. _____
2. _____
3. _____
4. _____
5. _____

FIVE THINGS I COULD BUY MYSELF
AS A TREAT – FOR UNDER $10
Samples: A pre-viewed video from the "sale bin" at the video store. A funny magnet to put on my refrigerator so I remember my victory each time I go for a snack. A new paperback novel.

1. _____
2. _____
3. _____
4. _____
5. _____

FIVE HEALTHY FOOD TREATS I COULD
USE FOR CELEBRATION "SUBSTITUTES" –
FOR AT LEAST $1/2$ THE CALORIES
Samples: A cereal bar for a jumbo, chewy, chocolate chip cookie. A banana instead of a banana ice-cream bar. A bag of low-fat, cheese-flavored baked chips instead of regular chips and cheese dip.

1. _____
2. _____
3. _____
4. _____
5. _____

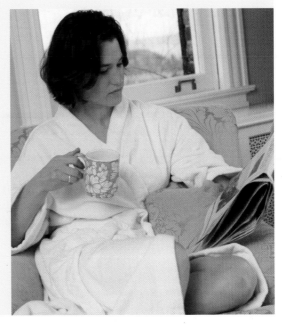

talk to your doctor. Most health experts say that to stay healthy, you should keep alcohol consumption to a moderate, infrequent level, such as one glass of wine or beer per day at the most. It's OK to incorporate the occasional glass of wine or beer as a part of your calories for the day. The key with alcohol consumption, as with other aspects of your quest, is moderation.

If you think you can stick to one serving, you might like to enjoy lower-fat or lower-calorie sweets or other treats once in a while. Take the time to search for healthier alternatives to your favorite high-calorie foods. Dried fruits or trail mixes can be very sweet and satisfying and, when eaten in small servings (such as a quarter of a cup), can be a healthy addition to your diet, adding fiber and important nutrients. Or, look for reduced-calorie versions of your favorite foods, such as low-fat frozen yogurt, reduced-fat cookies or fat-free pudding.

Take time to shop for groceries when and if you can. It's hard when you're in a rush to get home from work and cook dinner, or if you have the kids with you and they're screaming for the latest sugar-coated cereal.

If possible, take at least one grocery-shopping trip without the kids, and take some time to read the nutrition labels on the packages (we'll explain more about those labels in Chapter Four) to learn the caloric content and the serving sizes of various foods. Don't think because a food is "fat-free," "low-fat" or "reduced-calorie" that you should eat three times as much as the "serving size" on the label suggests.

Make a list of the healthy food items that you would like to buy in the future, foods that fit into your diet goals. That way, when you shop in the future – when you are in a rush – you will already know what items to grab quickly to stay within your healthy eating plan.

When you do celebrate with a treat, learn to savor what you are eating. Eat slowly and in a relaxed fashion. Sit down to eat a half-cup of frozen yogurt, eating each spoonful at a relaxed pace.

If you eat this way rather than shoveling the yogurt straight from the carton into your mouth in front of the wide-open freezer, you will eat less and enjoy the treat more.

Let's recap some of the things you have learned in this chapter:

- Try to find non-food alternatives for your celebrations. Make these things (or activities) that you really enjoy.

- Learn the recommended serving sizes of various foods and drinks so you can enjoy them in moderation.

- Consult your doctor, a nutritionist or a dietitian for professional guidance on what moderation means for you, and what particular problems you may have.

- Take time to shop for groceries when you can, so you can make the right decisions about what to buy, and so you can find healthier alternatives to your favorite high-calorie treats.

- When you do celebrate with a food treat, savor what you are eating. Eat slowly and in a relaxed fashion, so you enjoy what you are eating.

CHANGE the Way YOU EAT

Making small changes to what you eat every day and what you keep
in your pantry can help you cut calories and fat gradually.
That's the best way to keep excess calories out of your life for good!

As we learned earlier in this book, being overweight – or even worse, obese – is a major risk factor in developing many serious diseases and health problems, from arthritis to heart disease to diabetes.

What does it mean to have a "risk factor"? Simply, this means that you are putting yourself at greater risk for developing these serious diseases by being overweight – much greater risk than you would have for developing the problems if you were not overweight. This doesn't mean that you will never get a disease if you lose weight, but your chances of getting it are much, much lower.

When it comes to losing weight, you will have to set some goals for how much weight you wish to lose. In this chapter, we'll provide some general standards for healthy weights or other measurements, but we recommend that you consult your physician before setting any goals

or beginning any weight-loss or exercise program. By talking to your physician, you can review any particular health problems you have, your current weight, and any problems you may have with increasing your physical activity.

Set Some Weight-Loss Goals

If you think that you have some weight to lose, and if your doctor agrees, then together you should set some basic goals. Your weight-loss goals need to fit your personal situation. Every person is unique and has individual challenges associated with weight. Every person has a different body shape or style, lifestyle and medical history.

That is why we suggest that you set weight-loss goals only with the help of your doctor. Make an appointment to see your doctor, or bring up this issue at your next visit. We will provide some

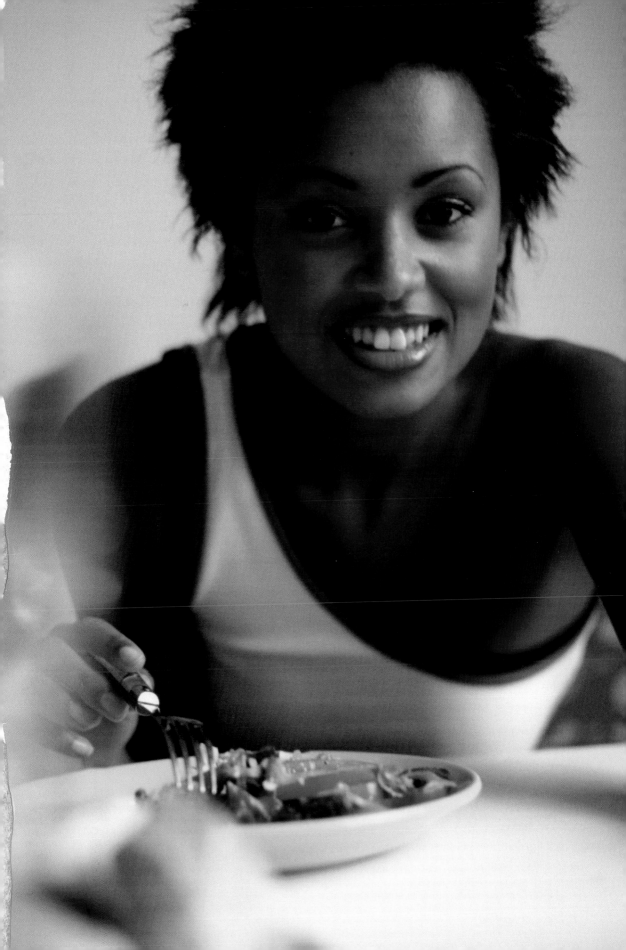

basic charts and measurements for healthy weights in this chapter. However, there are some more personalized tests that you can do with your doctor that will show you if you are overweight, and by how much.

With your doctor's help, you will set some basic goals for your weight-loss efforts. These goals might include:

• How much weight you should lose
• A range, in pounds, to aim for and to stay within once you achieve that level
• How long you should try this program, tracking your weight-loss efforts to determine your progress

When it comes to how long you should try any weight-loss effort, it really depends on you. The changes we suggest in this book and in this chapter are long-term changes. Permanent changes, in fact. We're suggesting that you set goals for yourself to make changes to your diet and eating habits that will last a lifetime. What you should aim to create is a nutritious, healthy, balanced diet. By eating this way, and by incorporating sensible physical activity into your lifestyle also, your weight will likely reduce as a result.

Losing weight by making gradual, healthy changes will be much easier than trying to make a drastic, short-term change to the way you eat. And this type of weight loss should be easier to maintain, because you will become accustomed to eating in a new way. It will seem natural to eat nutritiously.

As we said earlier, we are not suggesting that you give up eating chocolate for the rest of your life. What we are suggesting is that you find a desired weight range for yourself, and adopt the changes listed in this book as methods to help you stay within that range. Treating yourself to a sensible portion of chocolate (the key word being *sensible*) once in a while is fine, as long as you maintain a certain balance and don't burst through the top of your weight range.

Only you can discover the right formula for you and your lifestyle. What we will begin to learn here is that weight is related to a balance in your body – maintaining that balance is what healthy people do, and what you will learn to do by making these changes.

At the end of this chapter, we will help you set some goals for making healthy changes in your diet, and keeping an eye on your weight-loss progress. But first, it's important to explain more about nutrition, how the body processes food and how people might become overweight.

Unraveling the Mystery
of Weight Loss

How do you lose weight if you are overweight? And how do you know if you are overweight? First, let's explain a few important terms associated with weight loss.

OVERWEIGHT

According to the National Institutes of Health, being overweight means you have an excess amount of body weight compared to set standards. Excess weight may come from muscle, bone, fat and/or body water.

OBESE

Obesity means you have an abnormally high proportion of body fat. Therefore, a person can be overweight without being obese. A person who is a professional bodybuilder might have so much muscle that their actual weight on the scale is too high according to the standard for their age and height. But this person doesn't look over-weight, and may have no desire to lose weight.

Unless you are a bodybuilder, if you are over-weight, you may wish to lose weight to reduce your risk of developing the many diseases and health problems mentioned earlier. But losing weight, if you are overweight, can help you simply feel better. It can help you feel as if you have more energy. It can make it easier for you to be active. It can make it easier to fit into your clothes. We don't have to tell you the benefits of losing weight – you know them already.

BODY MASS INDEX (BMI) AND OTHER MEASUREMENTS OF WEIGHT

How can you determine if you are overweight? There are a wide variety of scales to determine how many calories you need to either maintain your weight or lose weight. Some scales, such as body mass index (BMI), are based on the proportion between your height and your weight. Others have to do with your percentage of body fat to body weight. (Think about the bodybuilder with the huge muscles – this person's muscles weigh a lot, so his weight is high, but his percentage of body fat is relatively low.) To measure your body fat, you can ask your doctor or other health-care professional to administer a skin fold caliper test or other fat-measurement test.

Body-mass index can help you see if your weight is in a range that is healthy in proportion to your height. To find your BMI, get out your calculator and do the following exercise:

1. Multiply your current weight in pounds by 704.5.

2. Then, divide this number by your height in inches.

3. Divide that result by your height in inches a second time.

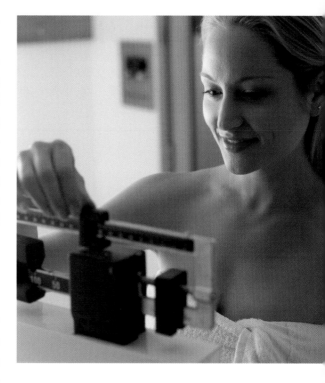

In other words, if Peggy is a 5'3" (63 inches) woman who weighs 145 pounds, her BMI is calculated by multiplying 145 by 704.5 (10,2152.5), then dividing that number by 63 (1,621.47), then dividing that number again by 63 = 25.7.

According to the National Institutes of Health, you are overweight if your BMI is between 25 and 29.9, and you are obese if your BMI is 30 or greater. So Peggy is slightly overweight according to the BMI index. To help you visualize where you fall in the spectrum of healthy and unhealthy levels, use the following two charts. The first chart will help you calculate your BMI (which you can also do with your calculator using the formula above) and the second chart will help you see if your BMI is OK or too high.

You may be surprised by what you find by either calculating your BMI or by checking where your weight falls on the healthy weight chart. You may find that your weight is quite a bit higher than the recommended level for a healthy weight.

Body Mass Index Chart

Body Weight (pounds)

Height (inches)	19	20	21	22	23	24	25	26	27	28	29	30	31	32	33	34	35
58	91	96	100	105	110	115	119	124	129	134	138	143	148	153	158	162	167
59	94	99	104	109	114	119	124	128	133	138	143	148	153	158	163	168	173
60	97	102	107	112	118	123	128	133	138	143	148	153	158	163	168	174	179
61	100	106	111	116	122	127	132	137	143	148	153	158	164	169	174	180	185
62	104	109	115	120	126	131	136	142	147	153	158	164	169	175	180	186	191
63	107	113	118	124	130	135	141	146	152	158	163	169	175	180	186	191	197
64	110	116	122	128	134	140	145	151	157	163	169	174	180	186	192	197	204
65	114	120	126	132	138	144	150	156	162	168	174	180	186	192	198	204	210
66	118	124	130	136	142	148	155	161	167	173	179	186	192	198	204	210	216
67	121	127	134	140	146	153	159	166	172	178	185	191	198	204	211	217	223
68	125	131	138	144	151	158	164	171	177	184	190	197	203	210	216	223	230
69	128	135	142	149	155	162	169	176	182	189	196	203	209	216	223	230	236
70	132	139	146	153	160	167	174	181	188	195	202	209	216	222	229	236	243
71	136	143	150	157	165	172	179	186	193	200	208	215	222	229	236	243	250
72	140	147	154	162	169	177	184	191	199	206	213	221	228	235	242	250	258
73	144	151	159	166	174	182	189	197	204	212	219	227	235	242	250	257	265
74	148	155	163	171	179	186	194	202	210	218	225	233	241	249	256	264	272
75	152	160	168	176	184	192	200	208	216	224	232	240	248	256	264	272	279
76	156	164	172	180	189	197	205	213	221	230	238	246	254	263	271	279	287

Clinical guidelines on the identification, evaluation and treatment of overweight and obesity in adults, National Institutes of Health, 1998.

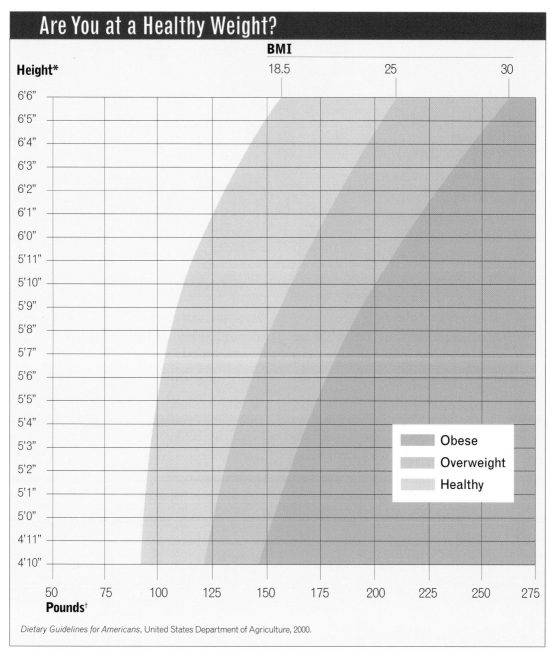

Are You at a Healthy Weight?

Dietary Guidelines for Americans, United States Department of Agriculture, 2000.

(These recommendations were developed by the United States Department of Agriculture, or USDA, which issues official reports on weight, eating and health called the "Dietary Guidelines for Americans." To view this report, log on to to www.ars.usda.gov/dgac.) Or you may discover that your weight is just slightly higher than it needs to be to be considered healthy.

However, there are drawbacks to using BMI or any other measurements of weight health. The best measurements for deciding if you are overweight or not are how you feel about yourself and what your doctor thinks. For example, maybe the jeans you used to wear all the time now feel tight and uncomfortable. Maybe you have noticed that the clothing you buy consistently is a size or two larger than the clothing you used to buy. These measurements may mean more to you than a BMI chart.

If you feel that you are overweight, if you have checked the above measurements and found that your weight is higher than the healthy range for your height, and if your doctor has told you that you might need to lose some weight, then it is time to make some changes in your diet and lifestyle to achieve that goal.

We've discussed some of the many risk factors associated with being overweight, and we have told you that being overweight can make you feel less energetic, more fatigued, less comfortable in social situations, less able to enjoy an active lifestyle. You know the reasons why you may wish to lose some weight. The question is...how do you do it and make it stick?

Many of us have tried to lose weight in the past, and found that this task is incredibly difficult. Often, we know what it takes to lose a few pounds – but it's hard to lose pounds and not gain them right back a few weeks or months later. Once you have gone through this discouraging cycle a few times (or more), you may feel that trying to lose weight is a no-win prospect. It just doesn't work! It's a waste of your time, you say.

But it is not impossible for most people to lose weight if they are overweight. You might have other health problems that make it difficult to make drastic changes to your diet or the way you prepare food, or in your ability to get

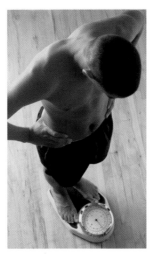

some physical exercise, a key factor in losing excess weight. But you can make some small changes that will help you, gradually and slowly, lose weight and keep it off.

Losing weight can be difficult for most people. There is no surprise in reading that statement. Why is it difficult? Because it involves things like commitment, determination, diligence and, above all, change! If losing weight were easy, there would not be so many weight-loss programs, products, supplements, fads, techniques and experts all around us, all with advertising that proclaims: This is the answer to your weight-loss problems!

Making Sense of All the "Diets"

You may have read about many "diets" or weight-loss programs that claim you can lose weight by cutting out one type of food or another from your diet. Every supermarket checkout aisle has a rack of magazines that advertise the "latest breakthrough" in weight loss, plans that claim you can "eat all you want" and still lose weight. You're probably fed up with reading these claims and skeptical about the prospects of real weight loss.

You may have friends who have lost dramatic amounts of weight on various popular plans. These programs are often called "elimination diets," because they suggest that you eliminate (or totally remove) a whole food group from your menu in order to eliminate excess fat from your body.

For instance, some weight-loss programs tell you to eliminate carbohydrates (the nutrient mostly found in bread, pasta, potatoes, carrots, corn, sugar and similar foods), because they claim that carbohydrates make your levels of blood insulin spike, making you hungry and craving more bread, pasta, starchy vegetables like potatoes, sweets, candy or similar foods.

Other weight-loss programs tell you to cut almost all the fats out of your diet, fats being nutrients found in oils, butter, many salad dressings, shortenings, nuts and avocadoes.

Some weight-loss programs push eating high amounts of proteins as the key to turning fat physiques into muscle-bound sculptures, proteins being nutrients found mostly in meat, fish, poultry, eggs, cheese and even beans.

The fact is that many of these weight-loss programs have complicated scientific explanations behind them. We won't go into the detailed theories of any of these programs, because each one could fill an entire book on its own. You've probably read many of these other books and have heard many of the various theories behind different methods of losing weight. Going into this topic further would only confuse you more.

Understand this: Some of these programs may work for you if your desire is to lose weight. But why do they work?

The reason these diets work is because they cut calories from your diet. These programs are known as calorie-deficient diets. There's that old word again – *calories* – but nobody has been using it for years, have they? Calorie has been replaced by other terms, such as carbohydrates, fats and proteins, right?

No – calories are still the key to any weight problem and any weight-loss strategy. Every food has a caloric value. You can read the caloric value of most foods by checking the nutrition label on the side of packages, or by looking up the value in calorie counter books available in most bookstores. No matter how you package the plan, the key to losing weight is calories, not fat or carbohydrates or any other nutrient.

In other words, you may cut out a lot of the fat in your diet by eating "fat-free" or "low-fat" foods in abundance. These foods can include things like celery or plain baked potatoes, but they can also include jellybeans, licorice sticks, fat-free chocolate pudding, fat-free turkey wieners and fat-free cheese. You might think that you could eat these foods in unlimited quantities, because these foods technically have little or no dietary fat. But all of

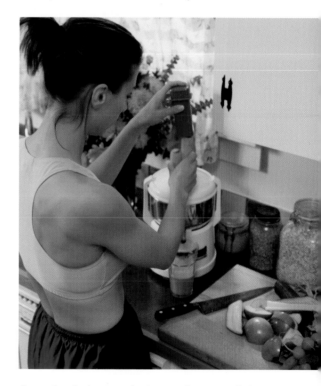

these foods have calories, and some of these foods are quite high in calories. By eating them in large amounts, you could be eating too many calories for your body's needs. And that leads to excess weight.

WHAT IS A CALORIE, ANYWAY?

All of this talk can be very confusing. What is a calorie? And why is this term important when we're talking about weight? A calorie is the amount or measurement of heat necessary to raise the temperature of one gram of water one degree on the Celsius scale.

Excuse me? What does this have to do with why my pants won't fit?

A calorie is also the unit of measurement of energy produced by food when it is oxidized, or used, in the body. Calories are like fuel for our bodies. We need them for our bodies to run. But if we pump more fuel into our bodies than we need for the amount of activity we do, the excess fuel just sits there. Your body will store this excess, unused fuel. It may store it as muscle, if you perform enough physical, muscle-building exercises such as weightlifting (remember the bodybuilder), or it may store it as fat.

You need to maintain a balance between the amount of calories you take in (food) and the amount of calories you use (exercise). You "burn" your body's fuel – calories – when you perform physical activities, and you also burn calories just by sitting still, breathing and living each day.

If you perform enough physical activity, you may increase the amount of calories (or energy units) you burn each day and raise the amount of calories (or energy units) you need each day. So a person who is physically active can eat more calories each day without gaining weight, because this person uses the fuel he or she pumps in, instead of storing it as fat. But we'll get into that more in Chapter Five.

Each person is different when it comes to the amount of calories he or she needs each day. The amount of calories a person needs for fuel varies according to age, height, gender, amount of daily physical activity and other factors. **On the next page is a chart to help you determine the amount of calories you will need to maintain a healthy or desirable weight.**

What's the Burn?

How many calories do you use by doing various exercises or ordinary activities? Here is a simple chart of some common workouts or activities and the approximate amount of calories burned during a 20-minute interval of moderate levels of these activities by a 150-pound person:

ACTION	CALORIES BURNED DURING 20 MINUTES
Dancing	120
Walking	80
Gardening	160
Cleaning	50
Aerobics	140
Driving	35
Cycling	160
Downhill Skiing	130
Weightlifting	140
Swimming	100
Tennis	120
Rowing	200
Golf	45

IF YOU EAT IT, WRITE IT DOWN

The best way to grasp how many calories per day you eat now, and how many you may be accustomed to eating, is to keep a food diary. Try this exercise for a week. Simply write down the foods you eat, 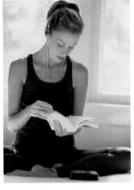 including portion size. Try to estimate the caloric content of each of these foods using a calorie counter book or by looking at the nutrition label on the packaging of the food. You may be surprised how easily calories add up!

Here are a few examples of common foods, a typical portion size and their approximate caloric values:

- American cheese, one slice: 70
- Apple, one medium: 80
- Apple juice, 8 fluid ounces: 120
- Bacon, two slices, cooked: 80
- Bologna, 1 oz.: 90
- Caesar salad, 10 ounces, with dressing: 520
- Carrot, fresh, one medium (7 inches long): 35
- Cheesecake, plain, 1/4 of 19-ounce cake: 330
- Cola, 8 fluid ounces: 100
- Frozen waffles, two: 220
- Hamburger roll: 130
- Macaroni and cheese, packaged dinner, 7.5 ounces: 260
- Milk, whole, 8 fluid ounces: 160
- Potato chips, 1 ounce: 150
- Pretzel twists, 1 ounce: 110

(These caloric values are measurements for a basic serving size. Check the nutrition information on the labels of your foods, or measure your servings, to determine caloric value.)

As you can see, the caloric value of different foods varies tremendously! And the amount of the food you can eat as a normal "portion" also varies quite a bit. It's important to rethink how you may look at what foods are "healthy," "nutritious" or "diet."

For instance, a Caesar salad, which is often coated with very highly caloric dressing, grated

How Many Calories
To Maintain Your Desirable Weight?

Desirable Weight (lbs.)	18-35 years	35-55 years	55-75 years
Women – Daily Maintenance Calories*			
99	1,700	1,500	1,300
110	1,850	1,650	1,400
121	2,000	1,750	1,550
128	2,100	1,900	1,600
132	2,150	1,950	1,650
143	2,300	2,050	1,800
154	2,400	2,150	1,850
165	2,550	2,300	1,950
Men – Daily Maintenance Calories*			
110	2,200	1,950	1,650
121	2,400	2,150	1,850
132	2,550	2,300	1,950
143	2,700	2,400	2,050
154	2,900	2,600	2,200
165	3,100	2,800	2,400
176	3,250	2,950	2,500
187	3,300	3,100	2,600

* Based on moderate activity. If your life is very active, add calories. If you lead a sedentary life, subtract calories. Prepared by the Food and Nutrition Board of the National Academy of Sciences National Research Council.

cheese and buttery croutons, can take up a large portion of your daily calorie budget. Does this mean you have to give up Caesar salads? Maybe not. You could budget the rest of your day's calories with low-calorie foods so you have room to indulge in your favorite salad. You could eat a much smaller portion of the salad to cut the calories you are eating. Or, you could make your own Caesar salad, with a lower calorie dressing, adding low-calorie fresh vegetables for crunch rather than buttery croutons.

Whatever you choose to eat, do your best to estimate the caloric value of the foods you consume and note them in your food diary. It won't be possible to know the exact caloric value of everything you eat, particularly when you eat in restaurants. But if you can estimate the calories you are eating, that will be a big help for you as you learn to budget calories wisely.

You can keep your food diary in a spiral notebook, a bound journal, on your home or work computer, or any way you choose. You can use the Changes Journal that we include the end of this book. It's important to find a method that is easy for you to access throughout the day and to remember to use. Try not to keep a mental record of what you ate and then write it down later – it's easy to block out a few chips here or a banana there.

Portion Control – The Best New Buzzword

As we learned earlier, even when you eat foods that are low in fat or relatively low in calories, the amount you eat is the most important factor. You will wish to keep the number of calories you eat per day within a healthy range, but you still want to eat a variety of foods for taste and

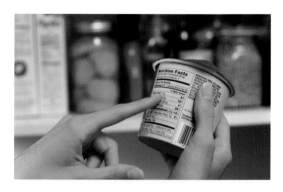

nutrition. And you will still want to eat enough to keep you satisfied. If you blow all your day's calories on a half of a chocolate layer cake (which sounds fun!), and then have to eat raw lettuce the rest of the day in order to stay within your healthy calorie range, that wouldn't be fun or possible to maintain on a daily basis.

You can eat almost any type of food and still stay within a healthy range of calories for the day. You simply have to decide how you will spend your budget of calories. Higher-calorie foods, such as french fries, will use up more of your budget than baked potato chips. If you want to budget your calories wisely, look at the sizes of the portions you are eating. Portion control is the most important diet buzzword you need to know. One of the biggest reasons so many Americans are overweight is that they have no concept of healthy food portions.

While it is important to consider the type of foods you are eating, it's really more important to look at the quantity of food that you eat. Many people know the right kinds of foods to eat. They know that baked chicken is more nutritious than fried chicken, for example. But many people have no concept of how much food is too much – and that misconception is a major contributing factor in their weight problems.

Part of the problem is an attitude inherent to American culture – we were all taught to clean our plates. Nobody is suggesting that you waste your food by throwing out what you don't eat. But it's OK to stop eating when you are satisfied, and to pack the rest away in a plastic, sealed container (or a "doggie bag" at a restaurant) to eat another time.

Many American restaurants, particularly those that serve "family-style" meals or fast-food restaurants, are capitalizing on the fact that their customers want value for their dollar. They do this by serving very large portions, meals that contain more calories than the average person probably needs at his or her meal. You think it is more cost-effective to order the double hamburger rather than the single hamburger, since the cost of the double is less than twice as much as the single burger. But do you need twice as many calories? Can your physical budget take the hit that suits your financial budget?

If the average adult female needs about 1,600 calories a day, do they need to eat a 1,200 calorie plate of pasta and meatballs at one meal? The answer is no – a portion size of pasta, for example, is one-half cup. But most of us have become used to eating larger and larger portions, and we feel deprived by going back to eating reasonable portions of food.

Many people underestimate how much they really eat at a typical meal. Like many Americans, you have come to expect large portions at restaurants, but instead of eating half the meal and taking the other half home (or sharing it with your dining partner), you eat the whole, gigantic portion. The result: You feel stuffed, sluggish and probably consume too many calories than you need in a day.

When it comes to eating, most people are driven by what they see, not by how they feel. Your hunger is driven by instinct. By putting

"Healthy Weights" for Women and Men

Height (without shoes)	Weight in pounds (without clothing)	
	Women	Men
6'4"	156-205	173-222
6'3"	152-200	168-216
6'2"	148-195	164-210
6'1"	144-189	159-205
6'0"	140-184	155-200
5'11"	136-179	151-194
5'10"	132-174	146-188
5'9"	129-169	142-183
5'8"	125-164	138-178
5'7"	121-160	134-172
5'6"	118-155	130-167
5'5"	114-150	126-162
5'4"	111-146	122-157
5'3"	107-141	119-152
5'2"	104-137	115-148
5'1"	101-132	111-143
5'0"	97-128	108-138

Source: *Report of the Dietary Guidelines Advisory Committee on the Dietary Guidelines for Americans*, USDA, 1990.

too much food in front of you, you will perceive this oversized portion as normal. If you change that habit, and start serving yourself smaller portions, you will perceive this smaller amount as a normal meal.

In one study, two groups of college students were asked, separately, to view and critique a movie. During the movie, each student was given a tub of popcorn to munch on. The first group was given a large tub of popcorn, and the second group was given a smaller tub, although each tub was full of popcorn. At the end of the movie each tub was weighed to see how much popcorn was consumed. The result: Neither group finished the tubs they were given, but the group with the larger tubs ate more popcorn. Most people will keep eating until they see that they have made some progress on finishing their portion – regardless of the size of that portion.

There are a few easy ways to determine healthy portion sizes for the various foods you eat.

On packaged foods, look at the "serving size" measurement on the nutrition label of the food's package. If you look on a box of cookies, and the "serving size" is two cookies, that means one portion is two cookies – not six cookies.

When following a recipe, look for how many "servings" the recipe makes. If the recipe says "serves four," that means that one portion is one fourth of the total amount of the food you prepare by following the ingredients and measurements in the recipe.

Get the Scoop on Serving Sizes

Do you know what you're eating? Below are some easy, visual cues for understanding healthy portion size.

So you ate a plateful of spaghetti for dinner

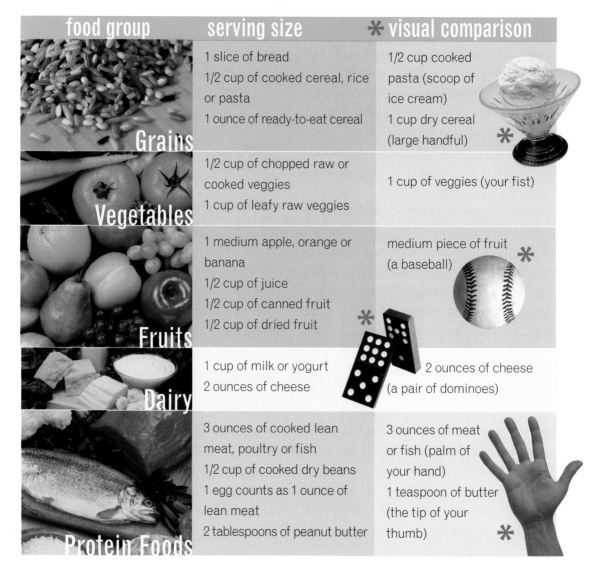

food group	serving size	＊ visual comparison
Grains	1 slice of bread 1/2 cup of cooked cereal, rice or pasta 1 ounce of ready-to-eat cereal	1/2 cup cooked pasta (scoop of ice cream) 1 cup dry cereal (large handful) ＊
Vegetables	1/2 cup of chopped raw or cooked veggies 1 cup of leafy raw veggies	1 cup of veggies (your fist)
Fruits	1 medium apple, orange or banana 1/2 cup of juice 1/2 cup of canned fruit 1/2 cup of dried fruit	medium piece of fruit (a baseball) ＊
Dairy	1 cup of milk or yogurt 2 ounces of cheese	2 ounces of cheese (a pair of dominoes)
Protein Foods	3 ounces of cooked lean meat, poultry or fish 1/2 cup of cooked dry beans 1 egg counts as 1 ounce of lean meat 2 tablespoons of peanut butter	3 ounces of meat or fish (palm of your hand) 1 teaspoon of butter (the tip of your thumb) ＊

and resisted the temptation to help yourself to seconds. Can you pat yourself on the back for eating one serving? Probably not. Minding food serving sizes is one of the keys to maintaining a healthy weight, but watching how much you eat can be a tricky business.

As we said, the dinner plates we buy for our kitchens seem to keep getting larger. And dining out these days makes it nearly impossible not to overeat: Meals at restaurants often contain enough meat and bread for an entire day.

Reward yourself if you're making progress downsizing the portions you typically eat, but challenge yourself to do better. It's easy to be a smarter "consumer." Learning to visualize servings is a useful skill, especially if you eat out a lot. Use the chart on page 52 to brush up on proper portion sizes and picture visual comparisons.

You may find it difficult to adjust your sense of a normal portion of food to reality. You may say, "I won't be satisfied with one cup of dry cereal." The key is to eat more slowly, to eat one bite at a time. Don't shovel your food into your mouth as if you were in an eating contest. Your body needs a little time to absorb your food so you don't feel so hungry.

It takes 20 to 30 minutes to feel a sense of fullness when you are eating. This sense of being satisfied or full tells you when to stop eating. That's why it's important to eat slowly. If you try to consume as much food as possible in 20 minutes, by the time your body catches up and feels satisfied, you are over-stuffed. You feel as if you couldn't eat another bite. Does that sound familiar?

Slow down when you eat. Eat one bite at a time, chew your food thoroughly and savor the taste of your food. That may be a hard habit to adopt, but you can make this one of your change-your-life goals.

SHOPPING FOR HEALTHY FOOD

Grocery shopping is a chore for most people. We are in a hurry, and we just want to get in the store and grab what we need so we can get home for dinner. So we often come home with bags full of high-calorie snack foods, frozen dinners and breakfast pastries.

It's difficult to find the time to shop wisely. It may help to make a list before you get in the store, and it also may help you to plan some menus for yourself or your family. This sounds like drudgery, but you probably do this in your mind already. What can I make for dinner tonight? I need this and this, and I have this in the freezer…so I'll make that into a meal!

If you really want to change your life, you have to be willing to alter some of your normal habits and your normal routine. So, once a week, perhaps when you are reviewing your journal, sit down and plan some meals for the next week. Take this meal plan with you when you shop so you can purchase the items you need. Or, if this is too much to figure out, just plan the next three days' meals. Or the next day's meals.

Think about how many calories you want to stay under for the day, and what foods might fit into that calorie budget. You should also try, as we said in Chapter Two, to include dairy foods, fruits and vegetables in your diet if possible, so you get enough of the nutrients that are important for health.

By sitting down for a few minutes and planning your meals for the next few days, you can keep to your nutrition goals and also stay within your calorie budget.

Later in this chapter, we'll look at the USDA's Food Pyramid, a good guideline for developing a healthy balance of foods and nutrients. By following this guideline, you will keep your intake of fats, carbohydrates, fiber and protein in balance, as well as get a proper amount of vitamins and minerals, essential elements for maintaining good health.

Here is an example of one day's menu plan with calories:

BREAKFAST:
Cereal and milk
Skim milk – 8 fluid ounces: 90 calories
Raisin bran (1 cup): 180 calories

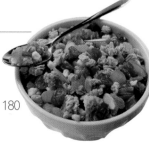

LUNCH:
Ham and Swiss cheese sandwich and pretzels
Rye bread – two slices: 180 calories
Baked ham – four ounces: 120 calories
Swiss cheese – one slice: 70 calories
Dijon mustard – 1 teaspoon: 5 calories
Leaf lettuce – 2 leaves: 5 calories
Pretzel twists – 1 ounce: 110 calories

SNACK:
Apple slices spread with peanut butter
One apple – medium: 80 calories
Peanut butter – two tablespoons: 190 calories
One cup of hot tea with lemon and non-calorie sweetener: 0 calories

DINNER:
Baked chicken breast with lemon-pepper seasoning, asparagus and baked potato
Baked chicken breast – whole: 160 calories
Baked in:
Two tablespoons fat-free creamy Italian

dressing: 35 calories
Lemon-pepper seasoning – 1 tsp.: 2 calories
Asparagus – 10 spears, steamed: 50 calories
Baked potato – 1 medium (5 ounces): 100 calories
Topped with:
Sour cream – light, 2 tbsp.: 40 calories
Herbs – dried: 0 calories

DESSERT:
Yogurt snack
One container (8 ounces) nonfat, sugar-free flavored yogurt, 100 calories

DAILY TOTAL: 1,517 CALORIES

By making meal plans such as this one, you can shop smarter when you go to the grocery store. You know you will need the items to make up this list. So you can shop for the items on your list, and try to stay away from items that don't fit into your meal plan. You can keep a separate list for your family's needs – particularly if your kids demand certain foods that don't fit into your healthy eating plan – and have the clerk bag those foods in separate bags. Make sure you let your family members know that you need these foods for your eating goals. Your spouse or kids might eat all the pretzels and leave you nothing but cheese puffs!

NUTRITION LABEL TIPS:
KNOW WHAT YOU'RE EATING
Almost every food in the supermarket that comes in a package has a label somewhere on the outside. This label is your best friend when it comes to figuring out sensible portion sizes,

nutritional value of foods and how many calories each portion contains.

Reading nutrition labels can be daunting if you have never looked at them before. But these labels offer you a variety of information about the food you are about to eat. How should you begin?

Read the "serving size" first to determine the portion of food that the information describes. Don't assume that one portion is the whole can or box!

Then, look at the nutrients and other dietary values in each serving. Use the following information to help you as you explore nutrition labels.

Keep an eye on the value of:

- Calories – particularly if you want to lose weight
- Saturated fat, total fat and cholesterol – particularly if you are a person at risk for heart disease, which may be linked to high cholesterol and high saturated-fat intake
- Sodium – particularly if you have high-blood pressure and need to control your sodium intake, an important factor in controlling high-blood pressure
- Sugars and carbohydrates – particularly if you have diabetes
- Fiber – particularly if you have problems with constipation or wish to reduce your risk of certain forms of cancer or heart disease
- Iron – particularly if you have problems with anemia

Fiber can be very important when you are trying to lose weight. Fiber is the indigestible part of many natural grains, fruits and vegetables. You may have heard fiber touted as being healthy because it adds "bulk" to your diet. This

means simply that foods rich in fiber (such as fresh fruits, whole-grain breads, fresh vegetables, popcorn) make you feel more full when you eat them. Fiber also helps your body eliminate waste more regularly and prevents constipation.

Too much fiber can be unhealthy, causing gas, stomach pains or loose stools, but eating a proper amount of fiber (estimated at 30 grams per day) can be very healthy and helpful to your weight-loss goals.

At first glance, the Nutrition Facts label on food packaging might look like a bunch of overwhelming numbers and charts and percentages. But when you know what you're looking at – and why it's there – you are one step closer to eating healthier. Here are some tips on getting the most from food labels.

- Learn the definition of claims on food labels. If a product calls itself "reduced fat," that means it has 25 percent less fat than the regular brand. "Light" means 50 percent less fat than the regular product, and "low-fat" means the product has 3 grams of fat per two-tablespoon serving. Compare the label on

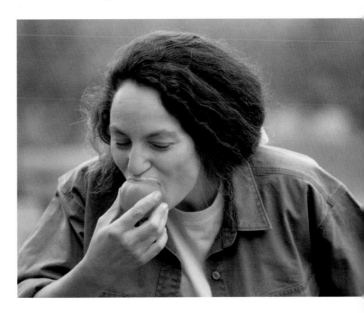

the lower-fat product to the regular one to see how much fat each lists.

- Pay attention to serving sizes. A serving size is based on the amount of food people typically eat. Be sure to compare the serving size of the product to how much you actually eat, and make sure you calculate the calories and other nutrient numbers accordingly.

- Note that Percent Daily Values vary. The daily values given on a label are based on a 2,000-calorie diet, which is a day's average for an adult male. Calorie requirements vary depending on gender, weight, age and activity level. You may not know how many calories you consume in a day, but you can still use the Percent Daily Values as a frame of reference. For example, try to limit your daily intake of fat, sodium, saturated fat and cholesterol to less than 100 percent of their daily value.

- Make sure the footnote's the same on all labels. At the bottom of the nutrition label is a list of how much, or how little, of some key nutrients you should eat each day, depending on whether you eat a 2,000-calorie or 2,500-calorie diet. This information is the same on every label, and is based on nutrition experts' advice. For example, the label states you should consume less than 65 grams of total fat if you eat 2,000 calories a day. That means that no more than 30 percent of your daily calories should come from fat. Some labels, if they are too small, will not include the full footnote. Remember: If you require less than the 2,000 calories per day that the label references, your daily requirements of certain nutrients, such as fats, may differ. Consult a registered dietitian or nutritionist for more information. But keeping your fat intake to no more than

30 percent of your daily caloric intake is a good rule of thumb.

- Read ingredients carefully. Ingredients, which are mandatory on food labels, are listed in descending order by weight, which gives you an idea of how much of an ingredient is present in the food in proportion to the product's overall weight. Reading ingredients ensures that you know if a food contains something you are allergic to, such as nuts, shellfish or wheat. The FDA also requires manufacturers to list food additives such as dyes or flavor enhancers. Also, beverages that claim to contain juice must list the total percentage of juice on the label.

- Note that sugar and protein do not have Percent Daily Values. No daily reference value has been established for sugar because the USDA has not made recommendations for the total amount of sugars to eat in a day. No protein daily value is needed unless the product claims it is high in protein or it's meant for children under 4 years old, because protein intake is not a public health concern for adults and children over 4. Therefore, when you see protein listed in the label, know that the nutrient is important for your body, but there are no specific recommendations on how much you should consume. Most scientists don't consider it a problem for most Americans to get enough protein, since the average American diet is quite high in protein.

For more information on nutrition labels on food, visit the USDA Web site, www.usda.gov. You can also call the FDA toll-free: 888/463-6332, or the food safety hotline toll-free: 800/332-4010. FDA food label information is at www.cfsan.fda.gov/label.html.

Eat Pyramid-Perfect –
It's Easier Than You Think!

How do you create a balance of healthy foods in your diet, getting enough carbohydrates, fats and protein, the right balance of vitamins and minerals, without too many calories? There is no simpler plan for eating a healthy, well-balanced diet than the one recommended by the USDA. To help you, the USDA created the Food Guide Pyramid. This is a handy visual guideline for eating a healthy diet. You can find the Food Guide Pyramid almost everywhere – look on your cereal box or other packaged foods. Simply follow the pyramid's at-a-glance daily advice: Eat more of the foods that form the pyramid's base and less of what's at the top. See the image on this page to learn more about the Food Guide Pyra-

mid. The food pyramid is a trusty guide for daily nutrition – one that doesn't require you to remember formulas or follow strict, food-eliminating menus, like fad diets do.

If you're trying to lose weight, fad diets are tempting: They may help you shed pounds quickly, as we learned, by cutting calories. But these diets often leave out important nutrients that you need for good health. You need carbohydrates, you need protein, you need fat, you need vitamins and minerals. Vitamins and minerals help prevent many types of diseases by preventing imbalances in your body. You may have heard about taking Vitamin C (found in oranges, for example) to help you fight a cold. By eating a healthy, balanced diet, you will eat a proper amount of all the essential nutrients.

Do you need to take vitamin and mineral

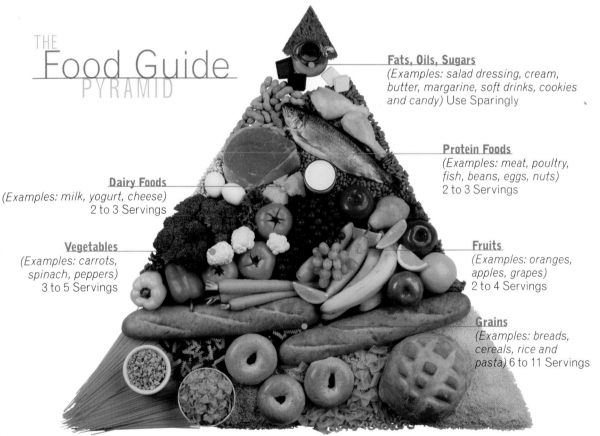

THE
Food Guide
PYRAMID

Fats, Oils, Sugars
(Examples: salad dressing, cream, butter, margarine, soft drinks, cookies and candy) Use Sparingly

Protein Foods
(Examples: meat, poultry, fish, beans, eggs, nuts) 2 to 3 Servings

Dairy Foods
(Examples: milk, yogurt, cheese) 2 to 3 Servings

Vegetables
(Examples: carrots, spinach, peppers) 3 to 5 Servings

Fruits
(Examples: oranges, apples, grapes) 2 to 4 Servings

Grains
(Examples: breads, cereals, rice and pasta) 6 to 11 Servings

supplements? If you eat a balanced diet, probably not. But you should ask your doctor if taking a multivitamin supplement is necessary for you. Some experts recommend that people who are trying to lose weight or cut calories should take a multivitamin supplement. Your doctor will be the best judge.

The USDA recommends eating a low-fat, high-fiber diet to maintain a desirable body weight and good health. We just learned why fiber helps you maintain regularity and feel satisfied when you eat. But why cut back on fat?

Fat is an important nutrient for keeping your body's organs functioning smoothly, but you only need small amounts. Fat is calorie-rich – 9 calories per gram versus 4 calories per gram for carbohydrate foods like whole-grain bread – so a little bit packs a lot of calories.

Fats are found in almost every food, but foods that are high in fats are very calorie-rich, dense foods like olive oil, butter, cream, cheese, red meat, nuts and avocadoes. The right kinds of fats, like olive oil, nuts and avocadoes, can be a healthy component of your diet in sensible proportions. Portion size is key when it comes to fats.

Keep in mind that all fats are not created equal. Saturated fats, such as those found in butter, ice cream or meat, can do damage to the coronary artery and lead to heart disease if eaten in too-high quantities. Unsaturated fats, monounsaturated fats and omega-3 fatty acids, such as those found in olive oil, nuts and fish, can be healthier and should be substituted when possible for saturated fats.

Therefore, a low-fat, high-fiber diet will keep the weight off and keep you satisfied, according to recent studies by the USDA. In other words, a traditional diet that's heavy on whole grains, fruits and veggies is the way to go.

Go Slow, Make Gradual Changes, Set Goals and Stick to Them

Losing weight is not an easy, instant change – you don't just wave a magic wand over your body and watch the excess flab disappear. Losing excess weight requires some willingness on your part to change the way you eat, the way you order dinner at a restaurant, the way you prepare food at home and the way you shop for food at the grocery store.

But we will offer you some guidelines for doing these things, some strategies to help you get through difficult situations, some methods for keeping yourself motivated, and then some terrific, healthy recipes to help you plan better meals and rethink the way you eat.

While losing weight does and should take time to be permanent, there are some simple changes you can make right now to improve the quality of your diet to make it more nutritious, lower in fat and calories. By making gradual changes to your diet, you can trim calories without feeling that you are deprived.

In the last chapter, we looked at how making one small change – substituting a cereal bar snack for a chocolate-covered ice-cream bar – could save thousands of calories a month in your diet. That's just one change! If you incorporated other small changes to what you eat, your calorie deficit would grow even more.

SNEAK IN GOOD FOOD – IT'S EASY

What's keeping you from eating better? Is your schedule so busy that you find yourself resorting to fast food or frozen pizzas for convenience? Do you find cooking difficult or too much of an effort? Whatever your barriers to nutrition may be, here are ways to improve your nutrition with very little effort. Try the simple tips on page 60.

Strong Bones, Strong Blood: Getting More Calcium and Iron

At your last checkup, did your doctor tell you to get more iron and calcium in your diet? Did you think, OK, I'll just eat cheeseburgers and milkshakes every day, because meat has iron and cheese and ice cream have calcium?

Many people are told to get more calcium and iron, whether through supplements (pills taken each day to add vitamins, minerals or hormones to your body) or certain foods. But they don't know why these two common nutrients are important for good nutrition and health. And they aren't sure which foods can put calcium and iron into their diets.

Calcium is important for building healthy bones throughout your life. It's especially important for children and adolescents to get enough calcium (about 1,200 mg per day) because their bones need strength as they grow. Adult men should get about 800 mg of calcium a day to keep their bones healthy, but grown women need calcium most of all — at least 1,200 mg if they're pregnant or nursing and 1,500 mg a day once they are past menopause. That's because women are most at risk for developing a disease called *osteoporosis*, in which bones become porous, brittle and highly prone to breaks.

To get more calcium in your diet, seek the following foods:

- Dairy foods (milk, yogurt, natural cheese, soy-based beverages with added calcium)
- Tofu made with calcium sulfate
- Breakfast cereals with added calcium
- Canned fish with soft bones, like sardines
- Fruit juice with added calcium
- Pudding made with milk
- Soup made with milk
- Dark-green, leafy vegetables like spinach, kale, collard or turnip greens

The good news for your "bottom line" is that you can eat the fat-free versions of yogurt, milk or pudding and still get all the calcium with none of the fat and less calories.

Iron is an important nutrient because iron helps distribute oxygen, necessary for life, to all parts of your body through your blood. People with too-low amounts of iron in their blood have a common condition known as *anemia*, which can be easily treated through iron supplements and adjustments to the diet. But anemia can become serious if left untreated, causing extreme fatigue and other problems. Women are especially prone to iron deficiency or anemia, so women need to make sure they get enough (adult males – 8 mg. per day; adult females – 18 mg. per day) iron in their diets.

To get more iron in your diet, seek the following foods:

- Shellfish, such as shrimp, clams, mussels, oysters or crab
- Cereals fortified with iron (check packages)
- Dark meat of turkey, without skin
- Spinach
- Lean cuts of meats, especially beef
- Enriched and whole-grain breads
- Sardines and anchovies
- Dry beans such as peas, black-eyed peas, lentils or kidney beans (cooked, of course)

- Buy whole-grain bread to use for your breakfast toast or lunchtime sandwich. You'll get more fiber from complex carbohydrates than from processed white and wheat breads.

- Sneak in fruits and veggies by stocking your refrigerator (both at home and at work) with ready-to-eat produce. Pre-cut fruit, broccoli florets, bagged baby carrots and celery sticks serve as easy snacks in between meals, or as welcome additions to your lunch or dinner plate. No chopping or cooking necessary.

- Add calcium by teaming veggies with easy-to-prepare yogurt dip. Make your own dip using plain, low-fat yogurt, chopped fresh herbs and a dash of lemon or lime juice.

If you are unable to eat dairy products because of lactose intolerance, the following foods are excellent sources of calcium that don't contain lactose: broccoli; bok choy; dried peas and beans; greens (kale, collard, mustard, turnip); canned salmon with soft bones; shrimp; calcium-enriched orange juice and almonds.

- Mix a handful of bagged lettuce with cherry or grape tomatoes for a quick salad to accompany a lunchtime sandwich or evening meal. To make your salad even healthier – without added hassle – try bagged spinach instead of lettuce. A nutrient superstar, spinach is chock-full of vitamins and minerals that help prevent cancer, heart disease and cataracts.

- Add protein to your salad the easy way by tossing in a handful of nuts, canned beans or lean meat or fish, like chicken or tuna. A sliced, hard-boiled egg also will boost your protein intake.

- When you do cook, aim for lasting results. Make a big pot of vegetable soup or a vegetarian casserole over the weekend and freeze it for later in the week. The extra effort will help you save time on hectic days.

- Avoid eating at fast-food restaurants. But if you must, try to make the healthiest choices. Opt for grilled meat (like a grilled chicken sandwich) instead of fried meat. Add lettuce and tomato to your sandwich. Hold the mayo. Substitute a side salad for french fries. Drink water or juice instead of soft drinks.

Now, you have some great information about why calories are so important to watch, how to determine what calorie range you need to stay within, what balance of foods make up a healthy diet, and how you can plan healthy meals, shop and cook. What's next? Get started by setting some goals for changing the way you eat.

As we showed you in Chapter Two, sit down and set some goals for changing the way you eat. Make them concrete, such as keeping within a sensible calorie range each day, eating according to the Food Pyramid, making menu plans and eating more fruits or vegetables. Use the sample goals and "first steps" provided in Chapter Two. If you like, make a contract with yourself (use the sample contract on p. 27) to follow these goals, sign it and stick to it as best as you can.

To help you keep track of what you are eating, write down what you eat in your Changes Journal. You will see where imbalances occur, and where you may need to reinforce your goals. If you try to divide your daily calories into three meals and don't leave some calories for snacks, you may get too hungry at certain times of day. You may feel deprived, and go way out of your daily calorie range by eating something unhealthy. Plan for snacks, and make sure you have them on hand when you need them. But write them down when you eat them!

Change Your Life
RECIPES

Try these great recipes as you begin changing the way you eat. These recipes are easy to prepare, add healthy nutrients to your diet and will help you plan healthy meals.

Each recipe gives you the suggested number of servings, indicating the proper portion size and the amount of calories and the following nutrients in each dish, so you can keep track of what you are eating and record the calories consumed in your Changes Journal:

- Fat
- Fiber
- Sodium
- Cholesterol

We suggest starting a file of healthy recipes to help you keep your diet full of variety and nutrition. You can tinker with the ingredients here – trying a different vegetable to substitute for another – or search for new healthy recipes in your local bookstore, online, at your local grocery store, or by asking your friends and neighbors. Don't be shy about sharing great ideas!

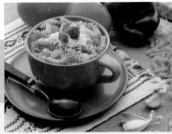

Appetizers

ARTICHOKE FRITTATA

A wonderful appetizer with lots of fresh-herb taste.

- 1 12-ounce jar marinated artichoke hearts
- 4 eggs, beaten
- 8 ounces small curd cottage cheese
- 1 small onion, chopped
- $1/8$ teaspoon rosemary
- $1/8$ teaspoon thyme
- $1/8$ teaspoon basil
- $1/8$ teaspoon marjoram

Preheat oven to 350 degrees.

- Drain artichokes, reserving 2 tablespoons marinade.
- Combine artichokes, reserved marinade, eggs, cottage cheese, onion and seasonings in a bowl; mix well. Spoon into greased 8-inch square baking dish.
- Bake at 350 degrees for 30 minutes or until set and light brown. Cut into 1-inch squares. Serves 16.

PER SERVING: Calories 56; Fat 4 g; Cholesterol 55 mg; Fiber 1 g; Sodium 186 mg

SHRIMP AND CRAB BALL

Impress your guests with this seafood delight.

- 8 ounces cream cheese, softened
- 1 teaspoon minced onion
- $1/4$ teaspoon Worcestershire sauce
- Salt, seasoned salt and garlic salt to taste
- 1 6-ounce package frozen cooked shrimp, thawed
- 1 7-ounce can crab meat, drained
- 1 8-ounce jar seafood cocktail sauce

- Combine cream cheese, onion, Worcestershire sauce and seasonings in small bowl; mix well. Chill in refrigerator.
- Add shrimp and crab meat; mix gently. Shape into a ball; place on serving plate.
- Spoon cocktail sauce over top. Serve with crackers. Serves 12.

PER SERVING: Calories 118; Fat 7 g; Cholesterol 63 mg; Fiber <1g; Sodium 282 mg

VEGETABLE DIP

An easy dip for all your favorite cut-up veggies
(or use with crackers).

    2 cups light mayonnaise

    2 cups light sour cream

    3 tablespoons grated onion

    3 tablespoons minced parsley

    3 tablespoons dillweed

    Seasoned salt to taste

- Combine mayonnaise, sour cream, onion, parsley, dillweed and seasoned salt in bowl; mix well.
- Chill, covered, for several hours to several days. Serve with fresh vegetables, such as baby carrots, bell pepper slices, cucumber sticks or broccoli florets. Serves 30.

PER SERVING: Calories 61; Fat 5 g; Cholesterol 10 mg; Fiber <1 g; Sodium 89 mg

GAZPACHO

A cool way to eat your vegetables!

    2 tomatoes, chopped

    2 cucumbers, chopped

    1 medium onion, chopped

    $1/2$ green bell pepper, chopped

    2 8-ounce cans tomato sauce

    2 10-ounce cans consommé

    $1/3$ cup red wine vinegar

    $1/4$ cup vegetable oil

    Pepper and garlic salt to taste

    Lemon juice to taste

- Combine tomatoes, cucumbers, onion and green pepper in bowl; mix well. Stir in remaining ingredients.
- Chill, covered, for 12 hours. Stir.
- Ladle into chilled soup bowls. Serves 6.

PER SERVING: Calories 158; Fat 10 g; Cholesterol 0 mg; Fiber 3 g; Sodium 955 mg

ITALIAN TORTELLINI SOUP

A tasty, filling soup for any season.

    4 14-ounce cans beef broth

    7 cups water

    1 pound sweet Italian sausage, cut into ?-inch pieces

    8 ounces frozen beef tortellini

    8 ounces frozen cheese tortellini

    8 ounces cabbage, shredded

    1 small green bell pepper, chopped

    1 zucchini, sliced

    1 small red onion, sliced

    1 14-ounce can whole tomatoes, crushed

    1 tablespoon chopped fresh basil

    Salt and freshly ground pepper to taste

    1 cup grated Parmesan cheese

- Bring all ingredients except Parmesan cheese to a boil in a stockpot; reduce heat. Simmer for 15 minutes.
- Ladle into soup bowls; sprinkle with cheese. Serves 20.

PER SERVING: Calories 137; Fat 6 g; Cholesterol 32 mg; Fiber 1 g; Sodium 897 mg

SUNFLOWER SALAD

Exotic mix of fruit and veggies.

    2 bananas, sliced

    1 cup thinly sliced celery

    1 cup shredded carrot

    $1/4$ cup golden raisins

    $1/2$ cup dry-roasted sunflower seeds

    2 tablespoons frozen orange juice concentrate

    1 tablespoon honey

    2 teaspoons lemon juice

    1 teaspoon poppy seeds

- Combine bananas, celery, carrot, raisins and sunflower seeds in bowl; mix well.
- Add mixture of oil, orange juice concentrate, honey, lemon juice and poppy seeds; toss to mix. Serves 6.

PER SERVING: Calories 187; Fat 10 g; Cholesterol 0 mg; Fiber 3 g; Sodium 26 mg

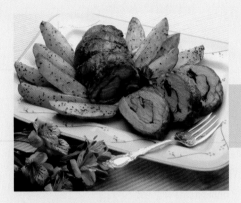

MARINATED PORK LOIN

A flavorful main course that will work nicely with almost any side dish.

   $^1/_2$ cup bottled lemon juice
   $^1/_4$ cup packed light brown sugar
   $^1/_4$ cup orange juice
   $^1/_4$ cup soy sauce
   $^1/_3$ cup vegetable oil
   1 tablespoon finely chopped fresh ginger
   $^1/_3$ cup sliced green onions
   2 $^1/_2$-pound pork tenderloins
   1 cup peach preserves

* Process lemon juice, brown sugar, orange juice and soy sauce in blender until smooth.
* Add oil gradually, blending constantly until smooth. Reserve $^1/_4$ cup of the marinade.
* Combine remaining marinade with ginger and green onions; pour over tenderloins in shallow dish.
* Marinate, covered, in refrigerator for 4 to 12 hours.
* Preheat oven to 450 degrees.
* Combine reserved marinade with preserves and melt, stirring frequently. Chill, covered, until serving time.
* Drain tenderloins, reserving marinade. Arrange on rack in foil-lined baking pan. Insert meat thermometer.
* Bake at 450 degrees for 10 minutes.
* Reduce oven temperature to 350 degrees and bake for 25 to 30 minutes or until 155 degrees on meat thermometer, basting frequently with reserved marinade. Chill. Cut into thin slices.
* Arrange sliced pork on serving platter. Serve with preserve sauce. Serves 16.

PER SERVING: Calories 192; Fat 7 g; Cholesterol 42 mg; Fiber <1 g; Sodium 297 mg

OVEN-FRIED CHICKEN

Delicious fried-chicken taste without all the fat and calories.

   6 pieces chicken, skinned
   $^2/_3$ cup baking mix
   1 $^1/_2$ teaspoons paprika
   $^1/_2$ teaspoon salt
   4 dashes of seasoning or herb blend, any type

* Preheat oven to 425 degrees.
* Rinse chicken and pat dry.
* Combine baking mix, paprika, salt and seasoning blend in sealable bag; shake to mix. Toss chicken 2 pieces at a time in seasoning mixture.
* Arrange on foil-lined baking sheet sprayed with non-stick cooking spray.
* Bake at 425 degrees for 35 to 40 minutes; turn chicken.
* Bake for 15 to 20 minutes or until chicken is cooked through. Serves 6.

PER SERVING: Calories 226; Fat 9 g; Cholesterol 81 mg; Fiber <1 g; Sodium 416 mg

CHICKEN AND SPINACH FETTUCCINI

A great, low fat, stick-to-your-ribs meal. Pair this higher-calorie main course with a fresh, green salad or steamed veggies sprinkled with lemon juice.

$1/2$ cup chopped onion
1 clove of garlic, minced
1 tablespoon margarine
2 tablespoons cornstarch
1 14-ounce can chicken broth
$1/4$ teaspoon basil
$1/2$ cup shredded mozzarella cheese
1 $1/2$ cups cooked chicken breast strips
4 ounces fresh spinach, chopped
1 12-ounce package spinach fettuccini, cooked, drained

- Saute onion and garlic in margarine in skillet for 5 minutes or until soft. Stir in cornstarch. Add broth and basil; mix well.
- Cook until thickened, stirring constantly. Add cheese. Heat until melted, stirring constantly. Add chicken and spinach; mix well.
- Cook for 1 minute or until heated through, stirring frequently. Spoon over hot cooked fettuccini. Serves 4.

PER SERVING: Calories 527; Fat 10 g; Cholesterol 57 mg; Fiber 3 g; Sodium 775 mg

OVEN-BARBECUED PORK CHOPS

A simple way to bring zing to a staple meat dish.

8 1-inch loin pork chops
Salt and pepper to taste
8 $1/4$-inch slices lemon
8 $1/4$-inch slices onion
$1/2$ cup packed brown sugar
1 8-ounce can tomato sauce

- Preheat oven to 325 degrees.
- Brown pork chops on both sides in skillet. Arrange in baking dish. Sprinkle with salt and pepper; top with onion and lemon slices.
- Pour mixture of brown sugar and tomato sauce over pork chops.
- Bake, covered, at 325 degrees for 1 hour, basting occasionally; remove cover.
- Bake for 15 minutes. Serves 8.

PER SERVING: Calories 225; Fat 8 g; Cholesterol 71 mg; Fiber 1 g; Sodium 233 mg

*Herb Complements for Pork
Complement the flavor of pork with the addition of coriander, cumin, garlic, ginger, savory or thyme.

MUSTARD-BAKED CHICKEN

Mustard adds heat and flavor to chicken without adding calories or fat. Experiment with different brands of mustard, but check labels to make sure there are no added calories!

6 skinless chicken breast halves
Salt and freshly ground pepper to taste
$1/2$ cup prepared mustard
2 tablespoons light brown sugar
1 $1/2$ cups bread crumbs

- Preheat oven to 400 degrees.
- Rinse chicken and pat dry. Season with salt and pepper. Place on rack in baking pan.
- Bake at 400 degrees for 10 to 15 minutes or until brown. Spread chicken with mixture of mustard and brown sugar; coat with bread crumbs.
- Bake for 20 minutes; turn chicken.
- Bake for 30 minutes or until chicken is cooked through. Serves 6.

PER SERVING: Calories 265; Fat 5 g; Cholesterol 72 mg; Fiber 2 g; Sodium 540 mg

HALIBUT STEAKS WITH THYME AND TOMATO SAUCE

This fresh fish is great paired with any vegetable or side dish, and the fragrance of thyme makes the meal a special event.

$1/2$ cup chopped onion

1 garlic clove, minced

2 tablespoons olive oil

6 tomatoes, peeled, seeded, coarsely chopped

$1/4$ teaspoon salt

$1/8$ teaspoon coarsely ground pepper

1 cup chopped fresh parsley

2 green onions with tops, chopped

1 tablespoon melted margarine

1 tablespoon thyme

6 1-inch fresh halibut steaks

Salt and pepper to taste

- Saute onion and garlic in 1 tablespoon olive oil in saucepan until soft. Stir in tomatoes, $1/4$ teaspoon salt and $1/2$ teaspoon pepper.

Bring to a boil; reduce heat.

- Simmer for 15 to 20 minutes or until of desired consistency, stirring frequently.
- Process tomato mixture in blender or food processor until pureed. Return mixture to saucepan. Stir in parsley. Reheat just before serving.
- Combine green onions, 1 tablespoon olive oil, margarine and thyme in bowl; mix well.
- Season halibut steaks with salt and pepper to taste. Arrange on grill rack 4 inches from coals.
- Grill over hot coals for 5 to 7 minutes. Turn steaks; brush with olive oil mixture. Grill for 3 to 5 minutes or until fish flakes easily.
- Spoon tomato sauce in center of dinner plates; top with halibut steaks. Garnish with sprigs of thyme. Serves 6.

PER SERVING: Calories 222; Fat 10 g; Cholesterol 37 mg; Fiber 3 g; Sodium 192 mg

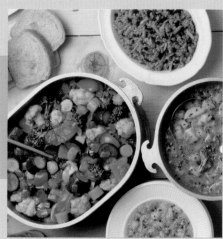

Side Dishes

GREEN BEANS WITH GARLIC

Garlic, the ancient bulb that is becoming a staple of contemporary cooking, adds tremendous flavor to fresh, green vegetables.

   3 pounds young tender green beans
   2 tablespoons extra-virgin olive oil
   6 garlic cloves, minced
   $1/4$ cup dry bread crumbs
   $1/4$ cup chopped flat-leaf parsley
   Salt and freshly ground pepper to taste
   $1/4$ cup margarine

- Steam green beans for 6 to 8 minutes or until tender-crisp; drain. Refresh in ice water; drain.
- Heat olive oil in nonstick skillet over low heat. Add garlic, bread crumbs, parsley and seasonings. Cook for 1 minute, stirring constantly.
- Add margarine. Cook until margarine melts. Add green beans. Cook until heated through, stirring constantly. Arrange in serving dish. Serves 12.

PER SERVING: Calories 100; Fat 6 g; Cholesterol 0 mg; Fiber 4 g; Sodium 70 mg

CARROT ROAST

Perfect for a winter feast, carrots are packed with nutrients like beta carotene and vitamin C.

   1 $1/2$ cups grated carrots
   2 tablespoons chopped onion

   1 cup cooked brown rice
   1 cup shredded cheese
   2 eggs, beaten (or egg substitute)
   1 tablespoon margarine, softened
   $1/2$ teaspoon salt
   Pepper to taste

- Preheat oven to 350 degrees.
- Combine all ingredients in bowl; mix well.
- Pour into greased 2-quart baking dish.
- Bake at 350 degrees for 45 minutes. Serves 8.

PER SERVING: Calories 127; Fat 7 g; Cholesterol 66 mg; Fiber 1 g, Sodium 376 mg

THREE-BEAN SALAD

The picnic classic returns as a great chilled comple-ment to chicken, sandwiches, cold roast beef or more.

   1 16-ounce can cut green beans, rinsed and drained
   1 16-ounce can cut yellow wax beans,
   rinsed and drained
   1 16-ounce can red kidney beans, rinsed
   and drained
   $1/4$ cup chopped green bell pepper
   1 medium onion, thinly sliced
   $1/2$ cup vinegar
   $1/3$ cup vegetable oil
   $1/2$ cup sugar

1 teaspoon salt

1 teaspoon pepper

- Combine beans, green pepper and onion in bowl; mix well. Stir in mixture of vinegar, oil, sugar, salt and pepper.
- Chill, covered, for 12 hours, stirring occasionally. Serves 10.

PER SERVING: Calories 166; Fat 8 g; Cholesterol 0 mg; Fiber 5 g; Sodium 596 mg

EGGPLANT CASSEROLE

Great as a hearty side dish, or try this dish as a vegetarian entrée paired with a salad or some gazpacho.

1 large eggplant, peeled, cubed

Salt to taste

1 tablespoon chopped onion

6 tablespoons margarine, softened

1 teaspoon salt

$1/4$ teaspoon pepper

$1/4$ teaspoon ground sage

1 cup cracker crumbs

1 cup cubed Cheddar cheese

2 eggs, beaten (or egg substitute)

1 cup skim milk

- Preheat oven to 350 degrees
- Cook eggplant in boiling salted water for 15 minutes; drain.
- Combine onion, margarine, 1 teaspoon salt, pepper, sage, cracker crumbs, cheese, eggs and milk in large bowl. Stir in eggplant. Spoon into greased 2-quart baking dish.
- Bake at 350 degrees for 45 minutes or until center rises. Serves 8.

PER SERVING: Calories 242; Fat 17 g; Cholesterol 71 mg; Fiber 3 g; sodium 640 mg

GINGERED ACORN SQUASH

An easy, hearty side dish with a zesty hint of exotic ginger.

2 small acorn squash

$1/4$ cup fresh orange juice

$1/2$ teaspoon ground ginger

$1/2$ teaspoon nutmeg

- Cut squash into halves. Remove and discard seeds. Cut a thin slice from the bottom of the squash so each vegetable will stand up straight in the dish.
- Arrange the squash in a shallow baking dish or pan.
- Place 1 tablespoon of orange juice in the cavity of each squash.
- Sprinkle with the ginger and nutmeg. Cover with foil.
- Bake the squash at 375 degrees for 1 to 1 $1/2$ hours or until tender. Let stand for 5 minutes before serving. Serves 4.

PER SERVING: Calories 121; Fat <1g; Cholesterol 0 mg; Fiber 9g; Sodium 8 mg.

BAKED ZUCCHINI

Easy to prepare, this dish has all the elements to make anyone in your family like vegetables.

3 cups thinly sliced zucchini

1 cup baking mix

$1/2$ cup grated Parmesan cheese

$1/2$ teaspoon Italian seasoning

$1/2$ teaspoon salt

2 tablespoons chopped parsley

1 cup chopped onion

1 clove of garlic, chopped

$1/2$ cup vegetable oil

4 eggs, lightly beaten

- Preheat oven to 350 degrees.
- Combine all ingredients in large bowl; mix well.
- Spread into greased 9x13-inch baking pan.
- Bake at 350 degrees for 25 minutes or until golden brown. Serves 10.

PER SERVING: Calories 210; Fat 16 g; Cholesterol 89 mg; Fiber 1 g; Sodium 372 mg

Breads & Desserts

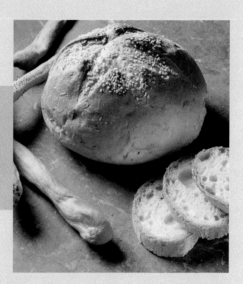

OAT CORN CAKES

These yummy cakes are a great breakfast when you're on the run — or top with fruit for a sweet, healthy treat after dinner.

   2 cups hot water

   2 tablespoons canola oil

   $^1/_3$ cup honey

   2 cups unrefined whole grain cornmeal

   2 cups oat flour

   1 teaspoon salt

- Preheat oven to 325 degrees.
- Combine hot water, canola oil and honey in bowl; mix well. Stir in mixture of cornmeal, oat flour and salt; mix well. Let stand for five to 10 minutes.
- Drop batter by $^1/_4$ cupfuls onto baking sheet sprayed with nonstick cooking spray; flatten with fork.
- Bake at 325 degrees for 30 minutes or until edges are light brown. Serves 15.

PER SERVING: Calories 160; Fat 2 g; Cholesterol 0 mg; Fiber 1 g; Sodium 143 mg

BANANA NUT BREAD

This classic American comfort food will take you back to your childhood.

   5 cups flour

   1 teaspoon salt

   1 teaspoon baking soda

   1 teaspoon baking powder

   2 cups mashed ripe bananas

   4 eggs

   2 cups sugar

   1 cup vegetable oil

   1 cup chopped pecans

- Mix flour, salt, baking soda and baking powder together.
- Beat bananas and eggs in mixing bowl. Add sugar and oil; mix well. Stir in dry ingredients just until moistened. Stir in pecans.
- Spoon into three foil-lined 5x9-inch loaf pans. Place in cold oven. Bake at 275 degrees for 1 $^1/_2$ hours. Serves 36.

PER SERVING: Calories 202; Fat 9 g; Cholesterol 24 mg; Fiber 1 g; Sodium 99 mg

PUMPKIN PIE

You love it at Thanksgiving, but this delicious dessert can be a special celebration treat year-round.

1 cup mashed cooked pumpkin

2 eggs

1 cup sugar

1 cup milk

1 teaspoon cinnamon

1 teaspoon nutmeg

$1/2$ teaspoon ground cloves

1 unbaked 9-inch pie shell

- Preheat oven to 350 degrees
- Combine pumpkin, eggs, sugar, milk, cinnamon, nutmeg and cloves in bowl; mix well. Spoon into pie shell.
- Bake at 350 degrees for 50 to 60 minutes or until set. Serves 8.

PER SERVING: Calories 259; Fat 10 g; Cholesterol 57 mg; Fiber 1 g; Sodium 153 mg

CHOCOLATE HAYSTACKS

Get the kids to help out with this fun dessert.

1 cup sugar

2 tablespoons baking cocoa

5 tablespoons margarine

$1/4$ cup milk

$1/4$ cup peanut butter

1 $1/2$ cups quick-cooking rolled oats

- Combine sugar, baking cocoa, margarine and milk in saucepan. Bring to a boil. Boil for 1 $1/2$ minutes, stirring to mix well. Remove from heat.
- Stir in peanut butter and oats. Drop by teaspoonfuls onto waxed paper. Let stand until cool. Serves 36.

PER SERVING: Calories 61; Fat 3 g; Cholesterol <1 mg; Fiber 1 g; Sodium 28 mg

CHOCOLATE-COFFEE PUDDING

Blending the tastes of coffee and chocolate, this dessert pairs great with a hot espresso.

$1/2$ cup firmly packed brown sugar

$1/4$ cup cornstarch

3 tablespoons unsweetened cocoa

1 tablespoon instant coffee granules

$1/8$ teaspoon salt

2 cups fat-free soy milk

2 ounces bittersweet chocolate, chopped

1 teaspoon vanilla extract

- Combine first 5 ingredients in a medium, heavy saucepan; stir well with a whisk.
- Gradually stir in soy milk; bring to a boil over medium heat, stirring constantly.
- Reduce heat and simmer 1 minute or until thick, stirring constantly.
- Remove from heat; add chopped chocolate, stirring until chocolate melts.
- Stir in vanilla.
- Pour about $1/2$ cup pudding into each of 4 dessert dishes; cover surface of pudding with plastic wrap. Chill at least 4 hours. Serves 4.

PER SERVING: Calories 261; Fat 4.8 g; Cholesterol 0 mg; Fiber 0.1 g; Sodium 149 mg

Use these recipes and more as you begin creating new menu plans and a new eating style for yourself. By following the Food Pyramid, eating sensible portion sizes and sticking to your daily calorie range, you will begin to lose weight. To help you lose weight, and to make you a more physically healthy, fit person, you should also set some goals to exercise. Exercise, as we learned at the beginning of this chapter, helps use up calories so you don't store them as fat on your body. Exercise will make you feel more energetic, flexible and strong. In Chapter Five, we'll look at some easy ways to change your life through exercise.

These recipes and more may be found in the cookbook *Help Yourself: Recipes and Resources from the Arthritis Foundation.* To order this book, call 800/207-8633 or log on to www.arthritis.org.

CHANGE the Way YOU THINK About EXERCISE

Exercise can help you burn more calories, lose weight and keep it off, feel more energetic and be more flexible. So why do so many people hate to do it? Here are some simple strategies to get limber, fit and strong.

There are at least one million reasons why people don't like to exercise. You must have a few to add to that vast number. Exercise is great for you, we know! But to many people, exercise is a time-consuming, difficult chore.

If you are going to lose weight, keep your weight under control once it is at a healthy level, and keep your body fit and strong to prevent diseases like arthritis or heart disease, you have to get some physical activity.

Regular exercise is important for everyone, no matter what your gender, age, current state of health or family medical history. There are documented reasons why exercise improves your health and can prevent serious disease. Exercise:

• Improves cardiovascular fitness so that your heart and lungs work as efficiently as possible;
• Keeps your muscles and bones strong to ward off conditions like osteoporosis and help your body support joints if you have arthritis;
• Prevents joints from becoming too stiff;
• Is a key component of any successful weight-loss program.

So exercise is vital to good health, and can help you lose weight and keep it off. The bad news: After reading why exercise is so important, you may still hate to exercise. The good news: We have some great suggestions for you on ways to get more exercise that are easy and fun to do. By making exercise more enjoyable – or at least easier and more convenient for your schedule – you will find that you can increase your fitness and

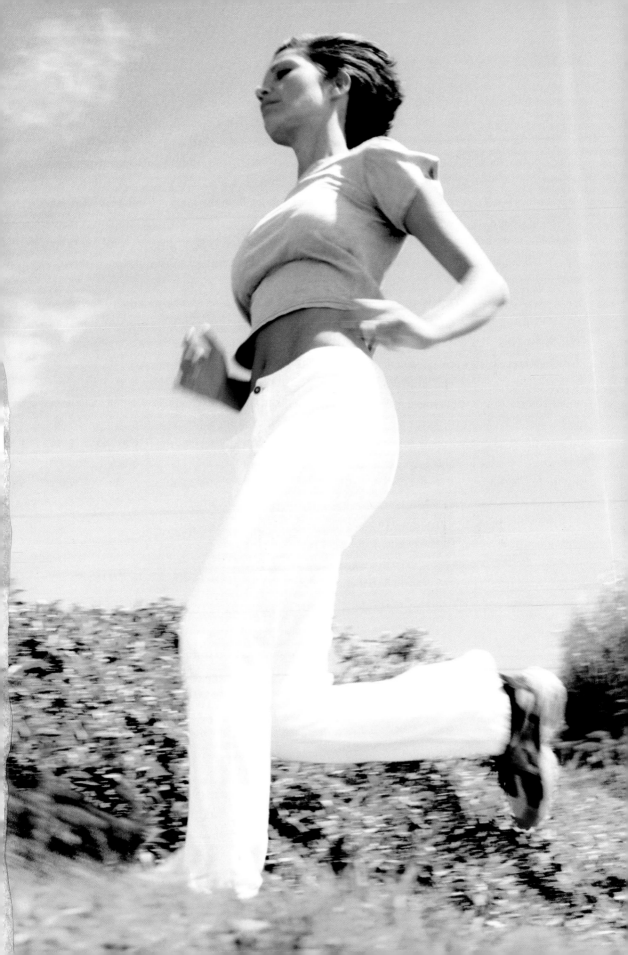

see great results in the way you look and feel.

In this chapter, we will look at the reasons you may have for not exercising – and why those excuses shouldn't keep you from getting active. You will learn how exercise benefits your body. You'll learn a little bit about the process of exercising – from burning calories to increasing your heart rate during your workout. You'll set some goals for getting exercise, and then learn the many easy, enjoyable ways you can get fit. It doesn't have to be a drudge!

Tossing Your Excuses Out the Door

Although exercise has proven benefits for your health – from helping you keep your weight under control to boosting your energy – many people just don't want to get off the couch and do something. They have many excuses for why they won't exercise or can't exercise. Is there a way to break through these excuses and find a reason why they can and should exercise?

Here are five of the most common excuses for getting out of exercise. The next time you hear yourself offering one of these excuses, try the reply offered here. This may get you out of your no-exercise rut and back into activity.

EXCUSE NUMBER ONE:

> *"I'm too busy to exercise, or I don't have time to exercise."*

Many people have busy lives today. We are a society of overextended people – we work long hours, we spend hours each week in traffic, we have endless obligations, we have children who engage in a different after-school activity each afternoon. Who has time to fit an exercise routine into such a busy schedule?

But exercise doesn't have to take up a 30-minute to 1-hour chunk of your day. New research is showing that you can break your exercise into 10- to 15-minute segments and get the same benefits. You might take a brisk 15-minute walk in the morning and after work, or try one of the many 15- to 20-minute exercise videotapes for a short-term aerobic workout (we'll explain that term later in this chapter).

You can also incorporate activity into your average daily activities by parking further from the entrance to a mall, taking the stairs instead of the elevator, doing yard work or cleaning the house to peppy music.

All of these simple activities don't take much time out of your normal schedule, and can have a significant impact on your fitness level. In addition, integrating more activity into your everyday routine may give you an energy boost, and encourage you to do more activity when you do have the time.

EXCUSE NUMBER TWO:

> *"I'm just lazy by nature."*

Aren't we all lazy when it comes to exercise? Who wouldn't prefer sitting in front of the TV with a bowl of popcorn to a 30-minute session on a stationary bike? Hopefully, when you find a type of exercise that you enjoy, and once you start increasing your fitness level, exercise won't seem so much like torture. But in the meantime, here are some tips for getting yourself motivated to exercise.

Find an exercise partner to encourage you to get moving. Having a partner for exercise, and setting an appointed time to get together to walk, swim or work out at the gym, will turn exercise into something more social and fun.

Ask around for a partner either in your neighborhood, at the local gym or online. You may look forward to exercising as a time to spend with your friend. You can encourage each other to stick to your exercise goals. And if another person depends on you to be present to exercise, you will be more inclined to do it. You won't want to let your friend down. So you may find you will be more inclined to take the time needed to work out.

Once you develop a regular "date" with your exercise partner (it can even be your spouse or another loved one), you will find you look forward to your workout.

EXCUSE NUMBER THREE:

> *"Exercise makes me sore."*

Some muscle soreness after exercise is normal, particularly when you are first getting started with an exercise routine. You may not have used those muscles in a while – or even known they were there! It is important to stretch before exercise, and to warm up and cool down properly (you'll find some suggestions for doing this in this chapter) so your muscles, tendons and ligaments are ready for your workout.

If you don't stretch your muscles before exercise, you increase your risk of a painful pulled muscle, and that injury can keep you from exercising at all for days.

If the exercise causes pain, stop and seek medical attention if needed. After a workout, soreness should only last about 24 hours. You can relieve this soreness with a warm shower and a mild analgesic such as *Tylenol*.

If the soreness lasts longer than 24 hours, you may have exercised too strenuously or too long.

You may need to adjust your exercise routine and try something shorter or less exerting. Try an organized, guided exercise class, such as those offered at local health clubs, community centers, YMCAs or in your neighborhood. If you are confused about what type of exercise to try, what level of exercise is right for you, or if you find that you do experience pain or extended periods of soreness when you exercise, consult your doctor.

EXCUSE NUMBER FOUR:

> *"I can't afford to join a gym."*

You don't have to purchase an expensive membership to a gym or health club to exercise. Buy a good pair of supportive walking shoes, map out a route and walk! You can try walking alone (make sure you walk in a safe, well-lit place) to have some cherished quiet time. Or, if you think you would be more motivated to walk with others, see if any of your friends or neighbors would like to start a walking club.

Another less expensive option is to purchase your own piece of exercise equipment. If you like riding a stationary bike at the gym, and don't use any other equipment there, it may be cheaper for you to purchase your own bike and keep it in your home. Shop around for a sturdy, low-priced

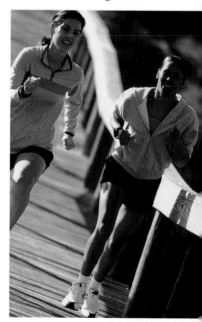

bike and test different equipment at the store before buying.

Some people prefer to work out in a gym setting, but find the high prices and, at times, required long-term membership contracts, prohibitive. There may be less expensive options. If you live in an apartment complex, there may be a workout room with various types of equipment available for you to use free of charge.

See if there is a YMCA, community center or church in your area that offers a workout facility – these may require a membership fee, but this fee is probably lower than those at a for-profit gym. Many community centers or churches offer workout classes, such as aerobics, step or spin classes, for a small fee. Do a little research, or ask your neighbors or your doctor for a recommendation.

EXCUSE NUMBER FIVE:

> *"I don't know how to start exercising."*

It can be difficult to get started if you don't do any exercise now, or if you have tried exercising in the past and given up. Making a good start to your exercise program is key for your long-term success. You want to try something that you think you may like to do – and that may not be the currently popular form of exercise that all your friends and neighbors do. If something seems too daunting – "I don't know if I could do that!" – then don't push yourself to try it. Luckily, there are many simple forms of exercise that are beneficial to your health.

Experts can help you find the right exercise, and exercise level, for you. Talk to your doctor. Seek guidance from well-trained professionals

in your area, including physical therapists, personal trainers or staff at your local gym or community center. Interview exercise staff to make sure they understand your personal needs. You may have certain physical problems that require you to develop a specific plan for developing your fitness. That doesn't mean you can't exercise at all – just that you need to find the right strategy for you.

When you go to your doctor for an annual exam, and he mentions that you need more exercise, speak up about your confusion and concern. Ask your doctor for a recommendation. Be prepared to try different exercise options. Understand that not every form of exercise will be right for you. If you can find one option – even something as simple as taking a walk – that's a great start! Get some fun, colorful workout clothes. Wearing your new outfit will motivate you to get out there and walk.

Face Your Doubts and Fears – and Move Forward!

You may have heard yourself say one or more of the excuses we just discussed. Perhaps you've never exercised regularly before. Or you're not sure how you will go from being a person who doesn't exercise at all to someone who exercises regularly. You may not even know where to begin!

If you are out of shape physically, or if you have a health condition such as arthritis, diabetes or fibromyalgia, you may be afraid that if you exercise, you will hurt your body. You might be afraid that you will push yourself too much if you exercise, or that you will experience pain. You might be afraid that if you exercise, you could damage your knees, your back, your muscles, your joints or other parts of your body. You may think that exercise is just too difficult

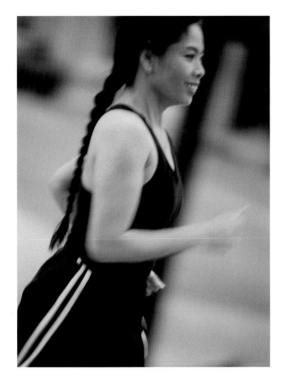

other people when it comes to how much you exercise, what type of exercise you do or how often you exercise. You need to find the type of exercises that suit your lifestyle and abilities. Here are a few tips to keep in mind:

- Start slowly.
- Choose activities you are comfortable with and capable of doing.
- Increase the levels of exertion or duration of exercise gradually, as you feel you are able to do.

Don't think of exercise as a chore – moving your body can be fun. Exercise can be just like play when you were a kid – it's recreation. Consider your "workouts" as "play-outs," time you carve out of each day to enjoy yourself and moving your body. Before you set exercise goals and get started on your new program, let's learn more about exercise's benefits.

Why Is Exercise So Good for You?

No matter who you are, some kind of exercise is good for your body. Research has shown that it can be especially helpful if you have certain

for someone like you, because you are too out of shape, or because at your age, you can no longer move your body the way you could earlier.

Put those thoughts out of your mind now! Here is the plain truth about exercise: Anyone can do it.

You don't have to be an athlete or even "in shape" to exercise or to benefit from the good things exercise does to your body. You don't have to be "good" at any particular sport or type of exercise to do it, do it regularly and improve your health. As you'll learn in this chapter, there are many different exercises for people with a wide range of abilities.

In Chapter Four, you learned that you shouldn't compare your weight or your body to that of a movie star or even to your neighbor down the street. The same goes for exercise. Exercise is not a competition. Don't compare yourself to

Benefits of Exercise

If you're not sure how exercise can help you, here's a sampling of ways exercise is good for you. Exercise can:

- keep your muscles strong
- improve your ability to do daily activities
- improve your overall health and fitness
- reduce feelings of depression
- give you more energy
- control your body weight
- give you an outlet for stress and tension
- help you sleep better
- improve your self-esteem and sense of well-being
- reduce fatigue

health conditions, such as arthritis, fibromyalgia or diabetes, or if you are at risk for developing heart disease. Exercising – even just a little bit – is an important way you can prevent some of these conditions and the negative effects of these conditions if you have them already.

Research has found that a modest exercise program will give your body the flexibility and stamina it needs to do the everyday activities you enjoy. In addition, exercise can boost your

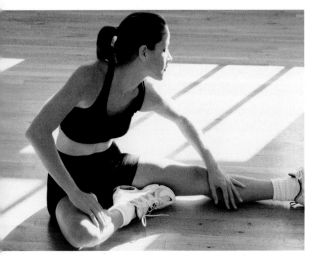

emotional well-being. Exercise can give you energy because it helps you sleep better. Sleep deprivation – a big term to describe the state when people are not getting enough sleep or are not getting quality sleep when they do sleep – is an increasingly common problem in America. When people don't get enough sleep, they can feel tired and distracted throughout the day, and they often see increased anxiety and crankiness. Their anxiety might be the reason they have trouble sleeping!

Exercise helps you work out your anxiety – think of punching a boxing bag to work out your frustrations. Exercise is an important part of your weight loss program, and can also help reduce pain, fatigue and depression.

WHAT IF YOU DON'T EXERCISE?

When you feel tired and out of shape, or if you are dealing with a health condition, the last thing you may want to do is get off your comfortable couch and move your body. But if you don't exercise and move your muscles and joints, you'll only feel worse.

Daily activities that were once just a little more difficult could become impossible for you to do if you don't keep your joints and muscles in shape through exercise. And not being able to do what you like to do – such as play catch with your son or go holiday shopping with your best friend at the local mall – can make you feel more limited, leading to lowered self-esteem and feelings of depression. It's a vicious cycle, but it's one that exercise can break for good.

How Do You Get Started On an Exercise Program?

Before starting any exercise program, you should consult your doctor. You need to discover which exercises are appropriate for your age, weight and physical ability, as well as any precautions you should take because of any medical conditions you may have.

Your doctor can recommend an exercise program or offer a referral to an exercise specialist, such as a physical therapist, a physiatrist (a medical doctor who specializes in exercise) or even a personal trainer. Ask your doctor if there are any specific activities or movements you should avoid.

For example, if you have pain in your knees, exercises that involve impact movements, such as step aerobics or jogging, may not be right for you. Your doctor, physical therapist or other health professional could recommend an appropriate alternative, such as water exercise. There is an exercise activity that is right for you – you just need to find it!

TAKING OFF AND STAYING MOTIVATED

Starting any exercise program can be intimidating, particularly if you've never been very active. Just keep in mind that you should start slowly. If you feel that you can't maintain a regular, strenuous workout at first, do what you can now. You can increase the duration and exertion level slowly.

For instance, if you like to take a short walk after work, try walking a little longer each time you walk. As you become stronger and your endurance increases, you will be able to exercise longer and more strenuously.

The toughest part of exercise, by far, is just getting started. But the effort you put into starting and maintaining a regular exercise program will pay off in huge rewards. You will experience more energy, better health, less fatigue and an improved emotional outlook.

Once you begin to exercise, you will find it easier each time you do your workout. Your body will become more conditioned. You may be surprised when you find that you look forward to exercising and can't do without it!

Here are some strategies that can help you stay motivated to continue your exercise program:

- Set a realistic exercise goal. Base these goals on some of the "first steps" you learned about in Chapter Two and the suggestions we offer in this chapter.
- Sign a contract with yourself. Write down what you plan to do and when you plan to do it. Have someone else "witness" the contract to help keep you motivated.
- Exercise at the same time each day if possible. Consistency helps exercise become a part

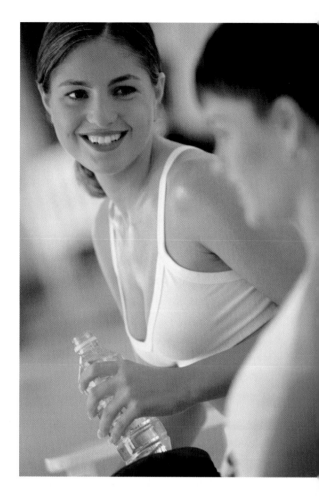

of your routine. Link the time to something else: For example, you can ride your stationary bike after you read the newspaper but before you take your shower.

- Stay in the habit. Do some exercise every day if you can. You don't have to do a whole "workout" every day if you are not able to – just make some effort to stay active, even if you just do some gentle stretching or flexibility exercises.
- Vary your routine. Some exercises, such as stretching or strengthening exercises are repetitive and can seem boring after a while. Try doing them to music or with a friend or family member.

- Evaluate your progress each month. You may be able to see the difference on your scale or feel it in your muscles.
- Celebrate your victories!

Exercise Stages:
Where Are You Going?

If you don't exercise at all – and many Americans are in this category, as we learned in Chapter One – making exercise a routine is a real challenge. You will have to propel yourself through a series of changes in your thinking about exercise. If you have always hated any kind of sports or physical activity, it will take a strong motivation to get started, and you will need to set small, incremental goals to keep you going.

If you have exercised sporadically in the past, but find it difficult to be consistent with exercise, you may just need to find the right activity for your lifestyle. Perhaps your schedule varies from day to day, making a jog after work or a swim class difficult to stick with. Or maybe you are bored with the type of exercise you have been trying, and need to find something new to spur your fitness quest.

Whatever your situation, you need to assess where you stand now so you can set goals for your physical fitness. The following section shows different stages of exercise readiness. By following the guidelines for each stage, you will progress to the higher stages until you reach a level of consistent physical activity and fitness.

STAGE 1
You Don't Understand
How Exercise Can Help You.

Weigh yourself. Have your posture or muscle strength checked at a health fair or screening pro-

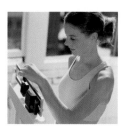

gram. Your doctor or other health-care professional can help you identify areas where you could use improvement and how you could benefit from exercise.

STAGE 2
You Know Exercise Is Good for You
and You're Thinking About Starting.

Now try to connect exercise with something you'd like to be able to do, like going on a hike with some friends from the neighborhood. View exercise as the way you will make these activities possible. Find friends or relatives who exercise regularly and ask them for suggestions for getting started.

STAGE 3
You're Getting Ready to Start an Exercise Program – But Don't Know How To Go About It.

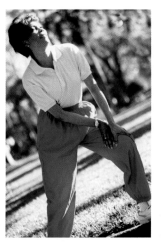

Choose an activity to try, but don't get discouraged if you don't like the first things you attempt. Learn proper stretching and technique so you can prevent muscle strain or injury, which in turn prevent you from doing more exercise. Talk to your doctor about an appropriate form of exercise for your physical condition. Make a plan by signing up for a class or sketching out a walking program. Set exercise goals for yourself.

STAGE 4

You've Started Exercising, but Sporadically.

Find ways to make exercise a daily habit. Map out your schedule each week to block off time for physical activity. Concentrate on good exercise techniques, such as warming up and cooling down, to prevent muscle strain that could discourage you to continue. Follow good form and gradually increase your exercise level as you work toward your goal.

STAGE 5

*You've Been Exercising for
Six Months or More.*

Great! Keep going and you will see measurable differences in the way you look and feel. Keep your body's fitness progressing by setting new exercise goals or trying new activities so you don't get bored.

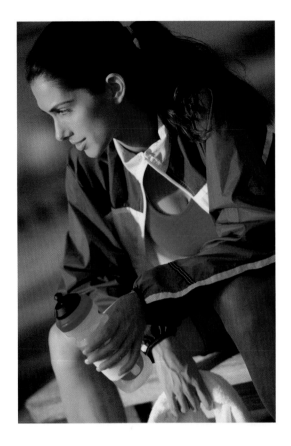

Mapping Your Progress:
Setting Exercise Goals

You have learned some important ways that exercise can help you get your weight under control and improve your health. In this chapter, you'll learn some simple strategies for increasing your fitness and making exercise enjoyable. Now, how will you really get started? You need to make a few decisions and set some exercise goals, so you can get off your couch and into some fun activity!

The first step is, as we said, talking to your doctor. With the guidance and information your doctor gives you, choose one form of exercise to try. (Later in this chapter, we'll show you a variety of exercise options to choose from.) Remember – if you don't like it or find it too difficult, you can always try something else! You

have not "failed." You simply don't like that particular activity. It's not for you, but something else will be. Just try something else. You don't have to explain your decision to anyone.

If you don't exercise at all, start with simple goals. A completely sedentary person (someone who spends most of their time sitting instead of moving) is not likely to go from couch to daily mountain biking. You would be asking for an injury and a huge feeling of disappointment.

Let's say you would like to try walking. Now, you need to make sure you have the right equipment you need to begin. Do you have good walking shoes and comfortable, flexible clothing? If you walk after dark, do you have reflective clothing so cars can spot you in their headlights?

OK. Now, where will you walk? Consider the options in your area. Are there some safe, well-lit places to walk? Do other people walk there, so that if you walk alone, you will be relatively safe? Are these places properly paved so you can walk with less risk of injury? Choose a good place to walk and a convenient time when you can walk on a regular basis.

Now, let's set some goals for developing a walking program (or whatever exercise you choose). To help you exercise consistently and effectively, we suggest that you create a contract, just like you learned in Chapter Two. Contracts allow you to spell out your goals. By writing your goals on a piece of paper, they become a little more concrete, a little more real. You are not just imagining yourself taking a walk or taking an exercise class. You are stating that you are going to try to do it!

Use the sample contract on page 27 or create your own. You might include rewards for each step of progress. All you need to do is create a written pledge of what you will do, how you will do it, where and when you will do it and how often you aim to do it. You can sign it yourself, or have your doctor, physical therapist or a friend act as a "witness."

Only you, with the possible assistance of your doctor, physical therapist or other professional, can set appropriate exercise goals for your needs. Only you can track your progress and determine if you are achieving your goals. So be your own coach!

In this chapter, you'll learn some ways to see if you are getting a good cardiovascular workout from your chosen activity and exertion level. You'll also learn some simple strategies and suggestions of various activities. But you need to determine what levels of activity and exertion are possible and productive for you.

For example, you decided you are going to try a walking routine. Your goal is to walk around your neighborhood for 30 minutes every day after work. Draw up the contract according to the form provided on page 80. Sign it. Post your contract on your refrigerator or bulletin board, or keep it in your Changes Journal.

It's important to keep a written record of your daily exercise activities, even if you only take a short walk or do nothing at all. As you learned in Chapter Three, keeping tabs on what you do and don't do will help you track your progress. Review the exercise entries in your Changes Journal at the end of each week, when you review your eating changes and plan your upcoming menus.

You will see if you are having trouble sticking to your goals. For example, you may see that walking after work is inconvenient, because you often have to work late. It may be easier to walk at lunchtime, or before work. Or, you may realize that you find daily walks boring – if you liked doing your activity, you might want to do it more consistently! Physical activity is the key to making all of your life changes more successful. So finding the right forms of exercise is also very important. You don't have to do only one activity – you can incorporate a variety of exercises into your life to make fitness a bit more interesting. In the following sections, we'll explore how to find the exercises you enjoy and offer suggestions of activities you may not have considered.

SO MANY CHOICES: PICKING EXERCISES FOR YOUR LIFESTYLE

When you're getting started on an exercise program – particularly if you have not been exercising at all – you may not know how or where to begin. There are so many ways to exercise – so many choices!

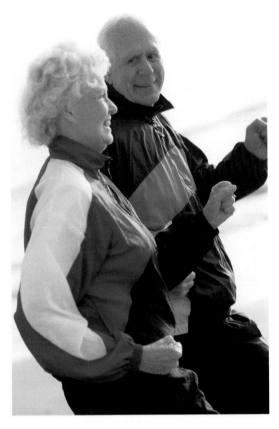

ing questions to narrow down your many exercise options and choose the one or more that are best for you:

- Do you find exercise more enjoyable when it is social – done with other people – or a solitary pursuit, a time to "get away" from work, family and other anxieties?
- Do you have the time and resources to participate in a team sport, such as a tennis league, golf foursome or softball team? Is there a community sports league in your area?
- Do you have the time and resources to participate in an organized exercise class, such as an aerobics, dance or karate class? Is there a class in your area?
- Do you enjoy exercising in a gym or health club environment or does this option turn you off?
- Do you prefer to work out in the morning, at lunch, in the evening or on the weekends? What activities fit into your schedule?

Almost any kind of activity that gets your body moving and your heart rate up (see the chart on page 84) can be "exercise." So how do you know what is right for you? Trial and error. Some activities will appeal to you, and some will not. You need to find something that is comfortable for you, and something that you think you can do on a regular basis. Some forms of exercise may be fun, such as playing in a tennis league. But what if you can't fit tennis into your busy work schedule? Don't be discouraged if you try something that doesn't pan out.

First, think about exercises you have tried in the past. What activities did you enjoy? What things did you despise? Think about the way you felt during these activities – not just physically but emotionally. Did you feel comfortable? Enthusiastic? Bored? Consider the follow-

Once you have considered these factors, here are some possible exercise choices for your situation and preferences:

- If you enjoy exercise in a social environment: Hiking club, walking with neighbors, tennis or golf foursome, water-exercise class, line dancing.
- If you enjoy exercise as a solitary pursuit: Walking, running, swimming laps, weight training, dance or aerobics to a videotape, yoga.
- If you enjoy team sports or competition: Softball, tennis, golf, ballroom dancing, flag football, kickboxing, cross-country running.
- If you feel you need an organized exercise class to motivate you: Aerobics, spinning, karate, yoga, step aerobics, Jazzercise™, dancing.
- If you like exercising in a gym or health club

environment: Kickboxing, aerobics, weight training, cardiovascular training (stationary bike, treadmill, stepper, elliptical trainer, etc.), yoga, tai chi.

As you can see, there are so many different types of exercise that choosing one is a tough task! Remember – you can try a few different exercises to see which one you enjoy the most. Or, you can do different activities on different days to stay motivated and excited about exercise. Working your body should be fun.

If you don't think you have the time, schedule, ability, motivation or resources to do a team sport or take an exercise class, don't worry. Exercise can be very simple and still be productive. The most important factor in developing an exercise routine is consistency. Whatever you do, you will want to aim for doing it on a regular basis. That way, you build your physical fitness steadily.

You should also try to be flexible. If you walk every other evening in your neighborhood, what will you do if it rains? Skip exercising altogether? Or could you walk at the mall instead? Exercise should be your goal, and you will learn to find ways to accomplish that goal despite challenges like weather, schedule changes and unexpected events.

GETTING THE RIGHT ELEMENTS IN YOUR PROGRAM

What you should aim for is developing an exercise routine. What does this mean? A good exercise routine incorporates some basic elements of physical fitness. Different forms of exercise can be combined to fulfill all of these requirements, adding some variety to your exercise. You may not be able to accomplish everything at once, but this routine is what you should aim for as your eventual goal.

Whatever exercises you choose, make sure that your routine contains the three basic parts of a complete fitness program:

- Flexibility
- Strengthening
- Aerobics

FLEXIBILITY OR RANGE-OF-MOTION EXERCISE

Flexibility exercise (also called range-of-motion or stretching exercise) is intended to help keep your muscles limber and your joints moving properly. These exercises can be thought of as the foundation of your exercise program, because flexibility is necessary for comfortable movement during all other forms of exercise and daily activities. These exercises also help reduce the risk of sprains and muscle strains when you participate in sports or other activities.

Flexibility exercises should be done gently and smoothly, usually every day. You may be familiar with this type of exercise as a "warm up," because these moves are usually recommended before performing any more vigorous type of exercise. Flexibility exercise can include

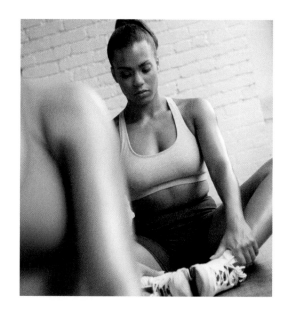

basic stretches, or more complex stretch-based routines such as yoga, tai chi or others.

If you haven't exercised in a while, start with flexibility exercise to begin your fitness program. Build up to a routine of 15 minutes of flexibility exercises. When you are able to do 15 continuous minutes, you should have the mobility and endurance needed to begin adding strengthening and aerobic exercise to your routine. Some sample flexibility exercises are included at the end of this chapter.

STRENGTHENING EXERCISE

Exercises that increase muscle strength and endurance are the second important component to improving your physical fitness. Strong muscles help absorb the shock of impact during activity – from intense sports to simple walk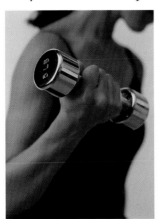ing around. Strong muscles support your many joints and help protect you from sports-related injuries. Strong muscles enable you to climb stairs, carry, lift and reach. Research has shown that strengthening muscles in the knee, hip and ankle led to improved balance in most people.

Strengthening exercises are also called resistance exercises. That's because these exercises make your muscles work harder by adding weight or resistance to movement. There are two types of strengthening exercises: isometric and isotonic exercises. In isometric exercises, you strengthen the muscles by tightening them without moving your joints. Isotonic exercises are just the opposite – you strengthen the muscles by moving your joints.

The goal of a good strengthening program is to overload your muscles just enough to get them to adapt to the extra work by becoming stronger. This can be done by adding hand-held or wrap-around weights, using elastic bands or simply using the weight of your body (such as in push-ups). You can also use weight machines or the resistance of water in pool exercises. If using handheld or strap-on weights, try using the lightest weights available first, then gradually add weight as you feel that the exercises are too easy to perform.

Don't overdo it, no matter what type of exercise you do. Don't overload your muscles with too much weight or resistance than they can handle, or you will risk getting a painful injury that will keep you from exercising at all. Don't worry if you feel you are moving slowly at first, or not exerting yourself very much. Just get into a routine of doing something active and you can increase the amount you exercise gradually. You'll get there!

AEROBIC EXERCISE

The term "aerobics" includes a wide variety of physical activities that make you sweat. Also known as endurance or cardiovascular exercise, aerobic exercises involve the body's large muscles in cadenced, continuous motions.

You may think that aerobics just means aerobic exercise classes, where an instructor leads you in a series of jumping and dancing motions set to a rhythmic musical beat. Or you may have tried doing aerobic exercise with a video. That kind of exercise is aerobic – but swimming, walking, hiking, biking, salsa dancing, using a step machine, playing tennis and even raking leaves are all aerobic exercises too.

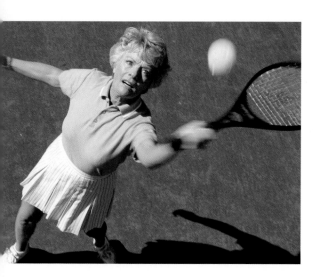

abetes, heart disease and high blood pressure. By making aerobic exercise a regular part of their routine, people may improve their endurance and sleep, reduce the effects of stress, strengthen bones and control weight.

You should include some type of aerobic exercise three to four times in your weekly fitness routine. You should aim to work within your target heart rate (see the chart below to find yours) for 30 minutes each session. If you find that you cannot exercise continuously for 30 minutes, progress to this level slowly. Begin by gradually increasing your activity for five minutes, continue with five minutes of activity in your recommended heart rate range, then decrease activity for five minutes. Once you have mastered this, you can increase the length of activity in your target range.

Aerobic exercise makes your heart, lungs, blood vessels and muscles work more efficiently. Aerobic exercise is crucial to achieving overall health. It reduces your risk of developing di-

Recommended Heart Rate Ranges Chart

AGE	HEART RATE RANGE (60% - 75% of Age-Predicted Maximum Heart Rate)	10-SECOND COUNT
25	117 – 146	19 – 24
30	114 – 143	19 – 24
35	111 – 139	18 – 23
40	108 – 135	18 – 23
45	105 – 131	17 – 22
50	102 – 128	17 – 21
55	99 – 124	16 – 21
60	96 – 120	16 – 20
65	93 – 116	15 – 19
70	90 – 113	15 – 19
75	87 – 109	14 – 18
80	84 – 105	14 – 18
85	81 – 101	13 – 17
90	78 – 98	13 – 16

KNOW YOUR TARGET HEART RATE

The chart on the opposite page shows you the recommended heart rate ranges for your exercise routine. You will have to measure how fast your heart is beating to know how much your body is working during your exercise. To monitor your intensity as you exercise, check your pulse about halfway into the most strenuous part of your walk. Here's how:

STEP 1

Press two fingers lightly on the inside of your wrist or the lower part of your neck.

STEP 2

Look at a watch or clock with a second hand and count the number of beats you feel in 10 seconds.

STEP 3

Multiply by six to get your heart rate per minute.

Your target heart rate when exercising should be 60 percent to 75 percent of your maximum heart rate (220 minus your age). For example, here's how the calculation is determined for a 60-year-old: 220 - 60 = 160; (160 x .60) = 96; (160 x .75) = 120. If your number is above the range, you're exercising too hard – slow down! If your rate is low and you feel OK, you can work harder. This way you reap the maximum aerobic benefits without causing harm to your health.

PERCEIVED EXERTION SCALE

During aerobic exercise, you should measure how hard you are working your heart and lungs to

What Is an Aerobic Exercise?

The term "aerobics" doesn't just mean organized exercise classes led by a *Spandex*-clad instructor, set to a disco beat. Any exercise that uses your large muscles in a continuous, rhythmic activity can be an aerobic workout. Some examples include walking, bicycling, aerobic dance and water aerobics. The signs that you are exercising at an aerobic conditioning level are:

* increased heart rate
* increased breathing rate
* increased body temperature or sweating

make sure you are exercising to the appropriate level of exertion. One way to do this is by using the Perceived Exertion Scale.

To rate how hard you are working, rate your exercise ability on a scale of zero (which is doing nothing) to 10 (working as hard as you possibly can so that you can't keep it up for more than a very short time). If you are new to exercising or you have significant limitations, begin at the very light to fairly light level (2-3). You should aim for moderate to hard intensity, or in the range of 4-7 on the scale.

0 - **nothing** (such as lying down)
1 - **very, very light** (almost nothing)
2 - **very light**
3 - **fairly light**
4 - **moderate** (still light but starting to work a little more)
5 - **moderate** (still comfortable but harder)
6 - **moderate** (getting to be somewhat hard)
7 - **somewhat hard**
8 - **hard**
9 - **very hard**
10 - **very, very hard** (couldn't do this for more than a few seconds)

The Talk Test

A simple way to tell if you're exercising at an appropriate level of exertion is the talk test. You should be able to carry on a conversation while exercising without feeling out of breath. If you're unable to talk, slow down a bit until you're working at a comfortable level.

As we learned earlier, there are countless ways to get aerobic exercise. You can explore different methods and find some that fit your preferences, abilities and schedule. Need some suggestions? Here are some simple strategies for getting a great cardiovascular workout.

WALKING

Walking is an excellent, easy aerobic exercise that almost everyone can do. Walking requires no special ability, and walking is inexpensive. You will only need to get a good pair of supportive walking or running shoes, and find a safe place and time to walk. You can walk in your neighborhood, at the park or mall, on a treadmill or on the track at your local high school.

The following suggested walking program may help you get your program started and advance it over time. When you can walk for a total of 10 minutes at a time (including warm up and cool down), follow this suggested progression chart to build your fitness program. If you can already walk for longer than 10 minutes at a time, enter the chart at your current level and progress from there.

More Great Ways To
Walk Your Way to Fitness!

In addition to its being one of the easiest forms of exercise – no equipment necessary – it's also one of the best for your health.

Walk fast enough and you can burn a load of calories; walk far enough and you can strengthen your bones, build stamina and help your lungs function more efficiently. Throw in reducing your risk of heart disease, lowering blood pressure and cholesterol, and curbing stress, and you've got a lot of great reasons to go for a walk.

Wherever you are in your quest for better health, whether just beginning or participating in regular exercise, there's a walking program for you. Here are four ways to approach one of the simplest forms of exercise. One of them is sure to be right for you.

DAILY WALKING

What is it? Daily walking is the kind you do all day long. In fact, according to the American Podiatric Medical Association, the average American takes 8,000 steps to 10,000 steps a day. While you may not consider walking to and from your car or from one end of the mall to the other real exercise, this type of walking can be just as effective as the other forms.

What's in it for you? People often overlook the physical benefits of everyday activities. Experts say that a little daily movement can add up. For example, walking grocery store aisles or doing housework can burn calories. The biggest benefit of daily walking is just starting somewhere. Before you can begin to think about how fast and how far you should walk, your focus should be on just moving. If you don't have a regular walking routine, then increasing your daily walking may be the easiest step.

What else? Walking is safe and puts less stress on the body than most forms of aerobic exercise.

Tips: Keep your head up and shoulders back. If you're always looking down, hanging your head and staring at your feet, you probably don't have the best walking posture. Good posture allows you to breathe correctly and can prevent misalignment of your back, neck and shoulders.

- Walk to lunch.
- Get off the bus or train one stop farther away than your usual stop.
- Take the stairs. (Surprisingly, descending stairs uses more energy than ascending.)

FITNESS WALKING

What is it? This type of walking – whether fast or not-so-fast – burns calories and improves

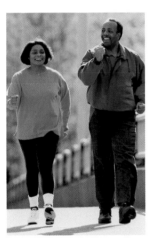

general health and fitness, particularly endurance. Try to build your distance, whether you walk on a treadmill, around a track or in the neighborhood. Start off with a few minutes a day and try to increase your time each session.

What's in it for you? Walking on a regular basis can help give you the energy and stamina you need to complete your daily activities, plus build bones and tone leg muscles.

What else? Walking is cheap. All you need is a good pair of shoes.

Tips: Find a walking buddy you can be accountable to. That way, it's harder to find an excuse to skip a day or two. Better yet, find a regular partner and an alternate for days when your main walking buddy is sick or unavailable.

- Drink plenty of water before, during and after your walk.
- Start slowly and progress gradually.
- Map out different routes with different distances both for variety and when you need to squeeze in a quick walk.

POWER WALKING

What is it? It's not running (which can be hard on the knees), it's not strolling (which is good for you, but doesn't burn many calories) and it should not be confused with race walking, a difficult and sometimes funny-looking type of walking. Power walking is walking at a fast pace to maintain cardiovascular health. You can do it anywhere – a track, around the neighborhood or on a treadmill.

What's in it for you? Power walking focuses on building cardiovascular health, which makes your heart stronger. Arthritis, age and other risk

Week #	Time Duration per Walking Session*	Frequency per Week
1	10 minutes	3-5 times
2	15 minutes	3-5 times
3	20 minutes	3-5 times
4	25 minutes	3-5 times
5	30 minutes	3-5 times
6	30-35 minutes	3-5 times
7	30-40 minutes	3-5 times
8	30-45 minutes	3-5 times
9	30-50 minutes	3-5 times

10 and onward: Keep your walks at 30-60 minutes per session, 3-5 times per week. Gradually increase your intensity until you are in the moderate range (if you are not doing so yet).

* Includes warm up and cool down, but not stretching.

factors you may have can affect heart health. This kind of walking weighs in as a total body workout, building bones and toning muscles.

What else? Walking at a brisk pace is an excellent way to burn calories.

Tips: The faster you walk, the greater your tendency to overstride, which can cause shin pain. Concentrate on taking shorter, quicker steps.

- Leave the headphones at home. You may not hear oncoming traffic or an angry dog.
- Warm up for a walk by first walking slowly for five to 10 minutes, then stretching. Cool down the same way.

HIKING

What is it? A hike is a walk that is off the pavement and into the woods, desert, mountains or other natural area. Call your local county or state park for information on walking trails.

What's in it for you? A hike is an excellent strengthening exercise. Many people don't view walking as a bone-building exercise, but it is. Because hiking involves walking on uneven surfaces, it also can be an excellent way of improving balance.

What else? Reducing stress is yet another benefit of hiking. Walking is one of the few exercises that allow you quiet time with yourself. When you're walking, particularly on a nature trail or anywhere outdoors, you can escape the daily hassles and stress of life.

Tips: Make sure you have the right shoes. How will you know? If your shoes are heavy, stiff (soles won't bend), more than a year old or too small, then it's time to replace them. Go to a shoe store, preferably one that specializes in walking shoes, and ask for a shoe that's right for hiking.

- Use a walking stick if you need extra support or balance.
- Take plenty of water with you.

WATER EXERCISE

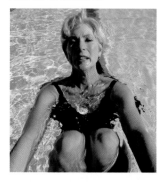

Water exercises such as swimming and exercising in warm water are fun and easy for anyone to do, even if you are overweight or out of shape. Water helps support your body while you move your joints through their full range of motion.

Swimming is highly recommended as an aerobic workout, because little stress is placed on your joints. Your local YMCA, community center or health club probably has information on water exercise classes in your area. Some communities offer water polo or other competitive sports done in water. Or, if you have access to a pool in your neighborhood, give swimming a try. Be safe by only swimming while others are around, however. On the following pages, you'll learn more about the pleasures of exercising in water, and get a great water workout to kick-start your fitness efforts.

Get in the Swim
With Water Exercise!

Sure, you'd love to exercise, but not at the risk of straining muscles or overexerting yourself to the point of pain and exhaustion. Or maybe you don't like to sweat, or find it embarrassing when you sweat during exercise. So why not do aquatic exercise, known to some people as water aerobics?

Exercise activities in the water are easy and effective. Water workouts are a fun, comfortable way to increase your flexibility and strength without risking injuries like muscle strains. The water's buoyancy and warmth is gentle and soothing while taking pressure off your knees, hips and back. Despite the fact that exercise in water feels easy and your body feels so light, water provides enough resistance to build serious muscle strength. Just look at the bodies of the synchronized swimmers at the Olympic Games!

If you're at Stage No. 1 in your exercise quest (see Chapter Two for information on health stages), just considering getting healthier, you may want to observe a water exercise class. If you're ready to take the plunge, sign up for an organized water exercise class at your local YMCA or gym, or try the following exercises on your own, with your doctor's approval.

Before you take the plunge, review these guidelines:

- Get a swimsuit that fits well and feels good. Don't worry about how you'll look in it, and don't compare yourself to other people in the class. Just make sure you are comfortable and can move freely in your suit.

- Keep your skin moisturized. Chlorine and warm water tend to dry out skin. Make sure you moisturize your skin regularly if you do water exercise. Consider wearing a bathing cap to protect your hair, and use a moisturizing shampoo or conditioner to keep hair from drying out due to chlorine. Note: Many pub-

Head-to-Toe **Water Workout**

Try these exercises at your community pool, in your hot tub or as part of an aquatic class.

Knee Lift

STEP 1: Stand with your left side against the pool wall.
STEP 2: Bend your right knee and bring your thigh parallel to the water's surface, or as high as you can. (Cup your hands behind your knee for extra support.)
STEP 3: Straighten your knee, lower your leg. Repeat on the left side.

Arm Circles

STEP 1: Raise both arms forward a few inches below water level. (Keep elbows straight.)
STEP 2: Make small circles (softball size) with your arms. Increase the circles to basketball size, then decrease.
STEP 3: Alternate between inward and outward circles. (Don't raise your arms out of the water or let them cross.)

Side Bend

STEP 1: Place your feet shoulder-width apart and relax your knees.

STEP 2: Bend slowly toward the right. Return to starting position and bend to the left. (Don't bend forward or twist or turn your trunk.)
STEP 3: You can try the exercise with your arms hanging at your sides, with your hand sliding down your thigh as you bend. Repeat on your left side.

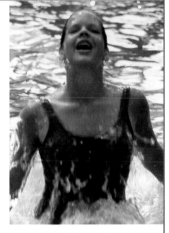

Ankle Bend

STEP 1: Place your hands on your hips or hold the side of the pool for support.
STEP 2: Bend your foot up, then down.
STEP 3: Repeat with your other foot.

lic pools ask swimmers to rinse off prior to entering the water to reduce oily lotion residue in the water. Make sure you moisturize after you get out of the pool, or after you take a post-exercise shower.

- Drink water. Just because you're surrounded by water doesn't mean you don't need to drink any. As with any exercise program, make sure you avoid dehydration by drinking water before, during and after exercising.

- Be fluid. The buoyancy of water protects your muscles and joints, but poor technique can still cause injury. Make sure your movements are smooth and controlled.

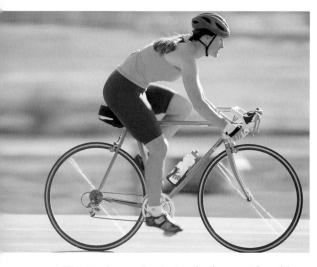

- Think of your feet. Beach shoes with rubber soles (no thongs or sandals) and other shoes made especially for water wear can protect your feet from rough pool floors. They can also prevent you from slipping as you walk around the pool, where surfaces can be wet and slick.

Other Great Aerobic Exercises

As we said, there are hundreds of ways to get your heart pumping and your body burning calories. Here are some suggestions for aerobic activities you might enjoy.

BICYCLING

Riding on a stationary, racing or mountain-style bicycle is a good way to get aerobic exercise. Stationary bikes let you get a great aerobic workout without placing much stress on your hips, knees or feet. Some stationary bicycles allow you to exercise your upper body as well.

Make sure you select a sturdy, comfortable, safe piece of equipment. You may wish to ask a physical therapist to recommend a bicycle. When beginning your biking routine, don't pedal faster than 5 to 10 miles per hour. As you become fitter, you can increase your speed and/or add resistance to your workout.

DANCING

Dancing activities, such as ballroom dancing, ballet, tap, jazz, square dancing, swing dancing, salsa dancing, country line dancing or disco dancing, can be a fun way to exercise, because dancing is almost always set to upbeat music. You can either dance alone or with a partner, or try forms of line dancing, in which you perform set dance steps in a line-up of fellow dancers.

Dancing can involve vigorous movements that raise the heart rate and increase cardiovascular fitness. Like other forms of exercise, dancing can also improve flexibility and muscle tone.

If you think your dance moves need some help, try a dance class, such as at dance schools, health clubs, community centers, houses of worship, schools or even at nightclubs. If you feel confident about your skills, you may just want to head out on the town with a partner or some friends and get moving! Make sure you wear comfortable clothes and shoes whenever you dance for exercise.

CARDIOVASCULAR EXERCISES

Sometimes known simply as "working out," a workout on basic cardiovascular gymnasium equipment – including treadmills, step machines, stationary bikes, elliptical trainers and more – is a popular, easy way to get aerobic exercise and to build muscle. Using these machines, whether at home or at a local gym, community center or YMCA, allows you to exercise in any weather. These machines generally are easy to use and allow you to create different exercise routines for yourself.

Do a little research before joining a gym or health club. Ask your friends and neighbors if they belong to a local club. Interview the club's staff before signing any membership contracts.

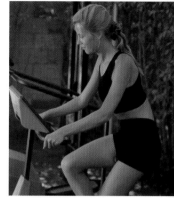

Ask the club if you can receive a short-term trial membership or some guest passes, so you can work out at the club a few times before deciding if you want to join.

You may decide that it's more convenient and cost-effective to buy a stationary bike or other exercise equipment. Try out several brands of equipment before making a purchase. Make sure you have a proper place in your home to put the equipment, with a sturdy pad or padded carpeting underneath.

Pains and Strains: Are You Doing Too Much?

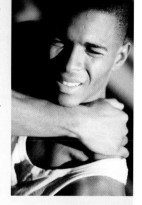

As we learned earlier in this chapter, you may find that on occasion, exercise makes you feel sore the next day. Some soreness is normal, because you are using muscles that may be out of good condition from lack of use. But you should know when you are exercising too much or in the wrong way, which can cause injury and pain.

Sore muscles are usually the result of overstretching muscles or overusing them by exercising following a long period of inactivity. This type of pain usually begins several hours after exercising and may continue for 24 to 36 hours. If you experience muscle soreness, you should spend more time doing flexibility or "warm-up" exercises before proceeding to more vigorous activity. You may want to scale back your program until your muscles become more accustomed to exercise, then gradually increase your workout. Review your exercise program with your doctor or therapist and modify it to avoid further injury to the joint. So exercise sensibly, but do exercise. You will feel better once you get in shape.

Watch for these signs that you may be doing too much and putting yourself at risk:

- increased pain that lasts for more than an hour after exercise
- increased feelings of weakness
- excessive tiredness
- decreased range of motion

Change Your Life

SAMPLE EXERCISES

for FLEXIBILITY and STRENGTHENING

Here are some sample exercises for general flexibility and strengthening that you can use in either a warm-up routine before aerobic exercise or to cool down after your workout. Note the precautions, if any, and choose the exercises that are best for you depending on which areas are painful. Always check with your doctor first before beginning any new exercise program or routine, and describe what form of exercise you are considering.

NECK EXERCISES

PURPOSE: Increase neck movement; relax neck and shoulder muscles; improve posture.

PRECAUTIONS: Do these slowly and smoothly. If you feel dizzy, stop the exercise. If you have had neck problems, check with your doctor before doing these exercises.

CHIN TUCKS. Pull your chin back as if to make a double chin. Keep your head straight – don't look down. Hold three seconds. Then raise your neck straight up as if someone was pulling straight up on your hair.

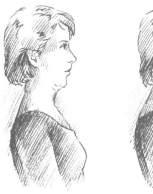

HEAD TURNS (ROTATION). Turn your head to look over your shoulder. Hold three seconds. Return to the center and then turn to look over your other shoulder. Hold three seconds. Repeat.

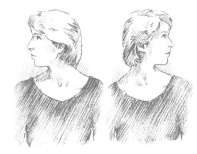

HEAD TILTS. Focus on an object in front of you. Tilt your head sideways toward your right shoulder. Hold three seconds. Return to the center and tilt toward your left shoulder. Hold three seconds. Do not twist head but continue to look forward. Do not raise your shoulder toward your ear.

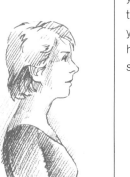
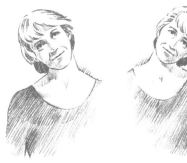

SHOULDER EXERCISES

PURPOSE: Increase mobility of the shoulder girdle (the bony structure that supports your upper limbs); strengthen muscles that raise shoulders; relax neck and shoulder muscles.

PRECAUTIONS: If the exercise increases any pain, stop and consult with your physician.

SHOULDER SHRUGS. (A) Raise one shoulder, lower it. Then raise the other shoulder. Be sure the first shoulder is completely relaxed and lowered before raising the other. (B) Raise both shoulders up toward the ears. Hold three seconds. Relax. Concentrate on completely relaxing shoulders as they come down. Do not tilt the head or body in either direction. Do not hunch your shoulders forward or pinch shoulder blades together.

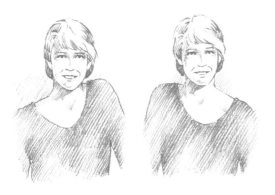

SHOULDER CIRCLES. Lift both shoulders up, move them forward, then down and back in a circling motion. Then lift both shoulders up, move them backward, then down and forward in a circling motion.

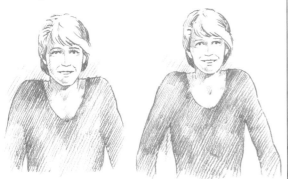

ARM EXERCISES (SHOULDERS AND ELBOWS)

PURPOSE: Increase shoulder and/or elbow motion; strengthen shoulder and/or elbow muscles; relax neck and shoulder muscles; improve posture.

PRECAUTIONS: If you have had shoulder or elbow surgery, check with your surgeon before doing these exercises. These exercises are not advised for people with significant shoulder joint damage, such as unstable joints or total cuff tears.

FORWARD ARM REACH. Raise one or both arms forward and upward as high as possible. Return to your starting position.

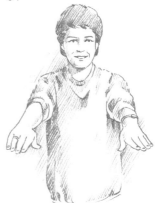

SELF BACK RUB. While seated, slide a few inches forward from the back of your chair. Sit up as straight as possible, do not round your shoulders. Place the back of your hands on your lower back. Slowly move them upward until you feel a stretch in your shoulders. Hold three seconds, then slide your hands back down. You can use one hand to help the other. Move within the limits of your pain. Do not force.

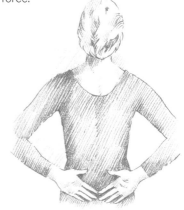

SHOULDER ROTATOR. Sit or stand as straight as possible. Reach up and place your hands on the back of your head. (If you cannot reach your head, place your arms in a "muscle man" position with elbows bent in a right angle and upper arm at shoulder level.) Take a deep breath in. As you breathe out, bring your elbows together in front of you. Slowly move elbows apart as you breathe in.

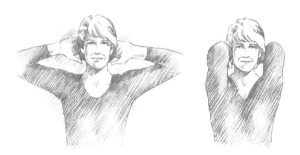

DOOR OPENER. Bend your elbows and hold them in to your sides. Your forearms should be parallel to the floor. Slowly turn forearms and palms to face the ceiling. Hold three seconds and then turn them slowly toward the floor.

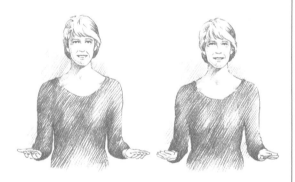

STRENGTHENING EXERCISES

PURPOSE: To build stronger muscles to help support joints better, make movement easier and to improve balance.

PRECAUTIONS: Avoid putting too much resistance or weight onto muscles at first. Resistance should be increased gradually to avoid muscle pulls, strains or injury.

BICEPS CURL. Sit in a chair, feet on the floor. Hold a one-pound weight in your right hand, letting your arm hang at your side. Bring your left arm across your chest, resting the back of your right arm on your left fist. Slowly bend your elbow, turning your right forearm toward the front of your shoulder. Your palm should be facing your shoulder. Pause, then lower your arm to the count of three. Repeat on the left side.

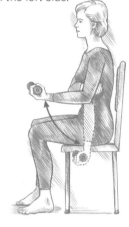

OVERHEAD TRICEPS. Sit in a chair, holding a one-pound weight in your right hand. Bring your right arm above your head, stopping when the inside of your elbow is above your right ear. Support your right upper arm with your left hand. Slowly bend your right elbow, lowering the weight to your right shoulder. Straighten your elbow to the count of three, pause, then lower it back to your shoulder. Repeat with the left arm.

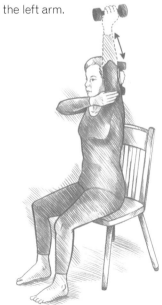

WRIST EXERCISES

PURPOSE: Increase wrist motion; strengthen wrist muscles.

PRECAUTION: If you have had wrist or elbow surgery, check with your doctor before doing this exercise. Stop if you feel any numbness or tingling.

WRIST BEND. If sitting, rest hands and forearms on thighs, table, or arms of chair. If standing, bend your elbows and hold hands in front of you, palms down. Lift up palms and fingers, keeping forearms flat. Hold three seconds. Relax.

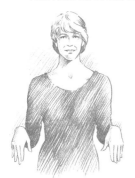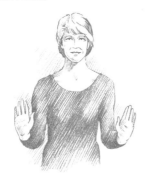

FINGER EXERCISES

PURPOSE: Increase finger motion; increase ability to grip and hold objects.

PRECAUTIONS: If the exercise causes finger or hand pain, stop and consult with your doctor.

THUMB BEND AND FINGER CURL. (A) With hands open and fingers relaxed, reach thumb across your palm and try to touch the base of your little finger. Hold three seconds. Stretch thumb back out to the other side as far as possible. (B) Make a loose fist by curling all your fingers into your palm. Keep your thumb out. Hold for three seconds. Then stretch out your fingers to straighten them.

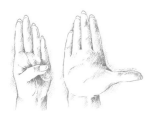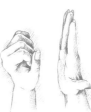

TRUNK EXERCISES

PURPOSE: Increase trunk flexibility; stretch and strengthen back and abdominal muscles.

PRECAUTIONS: If you have osteoporosis, back compression fracture, previous back surgery or a hip replacement, check with your doctor before doing these exercises. Do not bend your body forward or backward unless specifically told to do so. Move slowly and immediately stop any exercise that causes you back or neck pain.

SIDE BENDS. While standing, keep weight evenly on both hips with knees slightly bent. Lean toward the right and reach your fingers toward the floor. Hold three seconds. Return to center and repeat exercise toward the left. Do not lean forward or backward while bending, and do not twist the torso.

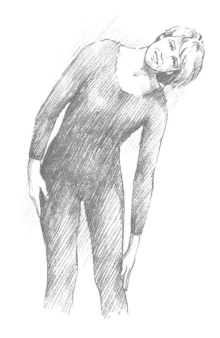

TRUNK TWIST. Place your hands on your hips, straight out to the side, crossed over your chest, or on opposite elbows. Twist your body around to look over your right shoulder. Hold three seconds. Return to the center and then twist to the left. Be sure you are twisting at the waist and not at your neck or hips. NOTE: Vary the exercise by holding a ball in front of or next to your body.

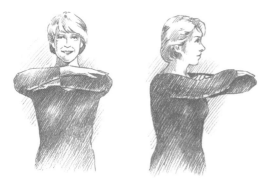

LOWER BODY EXERCISES

PURPOSE: Increase lower body strength; increase range of motion in hip, knee and ankle joints.

PRECAUTIONS: Check with your surgeon before doing these exercises if you have had hip, knee, ankle, foot or toe surgery, or any lower extremity joint replacement. Do not rotate the upper body unless specifically told to do so. When standing, avoid "locking" your knee joints by bending your knees slightly.

MARCH. Stand sideways to a chair and lightly grasp the back. If you feel unsteady, hold onto two chairs or face the back of the chair. Alternate lifting your legs up and down as if marching in place. Gradually try to lift knees higher and/or march faster.

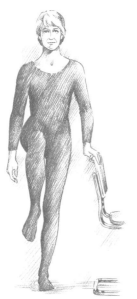

BACK KICK. Stand straight on one leg and lift the other leg behind you. Hold three seconds. Try to keep your leg straight as you move it backward. Motion should occur only in the hip (not waist). Do not lean forward – keep your upper body straight. NOTE: You can add resistance by using a large rubber exercise band around ankles.

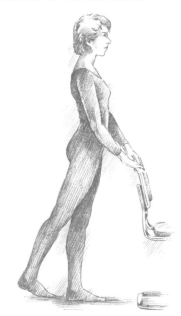

SIDE LEG KICK. Stand near a chair, holding it for support. Stand on one leg and lift the other leg out to the side. Hold three seconds and return your leg to the floor. Only move your leg at the top – don't lean toward the chair. Alternate legs.

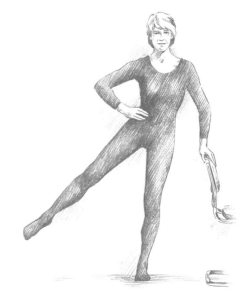

HIP TURNS. Stand with legs slightly apart, with your weight on one leg and the heel of your other foot lightly touching the floor. Rotate your whole leg from the hip so that toes and knee point in and then out. Don't rotate your body – keep chest and shoulders facing forward. NOTE: If you have difficulty putting weight on one leg, you can also do this exercise by sitting at the edge of a chair with your legs extended straight in front and with your heels resting on the floor.

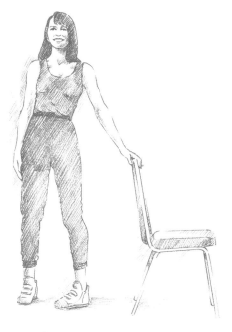

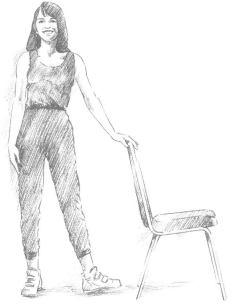

SKIER'S SQUAT (QUADRICEPS STRENGTHENER). Stand behind a chair with your hands lightly resting on top of chair for support. Keep your feet flat on the floor. Keeping your back straight, slowly bend your knees to lower your body a few inches. Hold for three to six seconds, then slowly return to an upright position. Don't allow your knees to go past your toes.

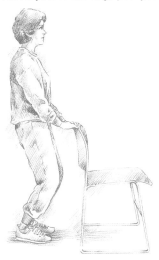

TIPTOE. Face the back of a chair and rest your hands on it. Rise up and stand on your toes. Hold three seconds, then return to the flat position. Try to keep your knees straight (but not locked). Now stand on your heels, raising your toes and front part of your foot off the ground. NOTE: You can do this exercise one foot at a time.

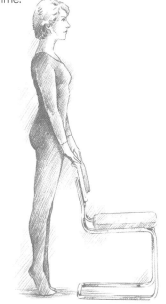

CALF STRETCH. Hold lightly to the back of a chair. Bend the knee of the leg you are not stretching so that it almost touches the chair. Put the leg to be stretched behind you, keeping both feet flat on the floor. Lean forward gently, keeping your back knee straight.

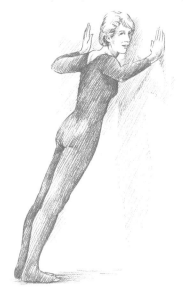

CHEST STRETCH. Stand about two to three feet away from a wall and place your hands or forearms on the wall at shoulder height. Lean forward, leading with your hips. Keep your knees straight and your head back. Hold this position for five to 10 seconds, then push back to starting position. To feel more stretch, place your hands farther apart.

THIGH FIRMER AND KNEE STRETCH. Sit on the edge of your chair or lie on your back with your legs stretched out in front and your heels resting on the floor. Tighten the muscle that runs across the front of the knee by pulling your toes toward your head. Push the back of the knee down toward the floor so you also feel a stretch at the back of your knee and ankle. For a greater stretch, put your heel on a footstool and lean forward as you pull your toes toward your head.

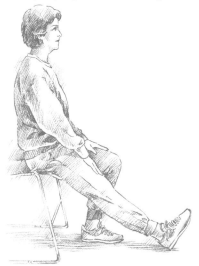

KNEE EXTENSION. Sit in a chair, your feet shoulder-width apart, knees directly above them. Put a towel under your knees for padding. With your hands on your thighs, raise your right leg to the count of three until your knee is straight (but not locked). Pause, then lower your leg to the count of three. Repeat on the left side.

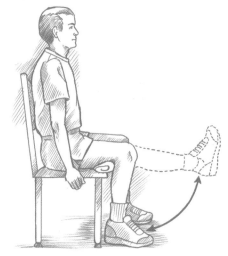

EXERCISES FOR THE POOL

If you have access to a swimming pool, try these moves specifically designed for the water. Many people find exercising in water easier, and it's also fun!

LEG SWING (HIP FLEXION/EXTENSION). Stand with one side against the pool wall, and hold on for balance. Perform slowly. Bring your thigh parallel to the water surface as high as is comfortable. Lower your leg. Gently swing your leg behind you. Repeat with other side.

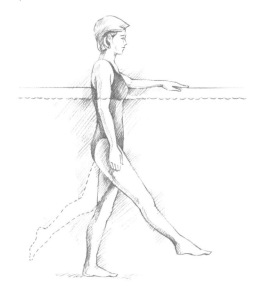

WALKING. Walk normally across or in a circle in the pool. Swing your arms as you walk. Wearing water shoes or sneakers is helpful.

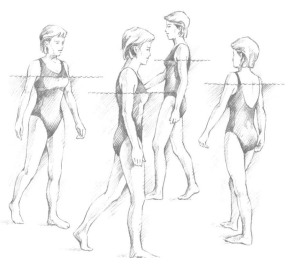

KNEE LIFT (HIP AND KNEE FLEXION/EXTENSION). Stand with one side against the pool wall. Bend your knee, bringing your thigh parallel to the water's surface as high as is comfortable. Cup one hand behind your knee if your leg needs extra support. Straighten your knee and then lower your leg, keeping the knee straight. Keep your ankles and toes relaxed. Repeat on the other side.

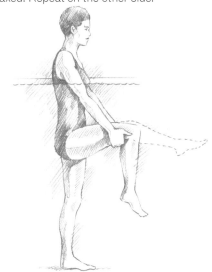

CALF STRETCH. Stand with your side toward the wall, and place your hand on the wall for balance. Stand straight with your legs slightly apart and with one leg ahead of the other. Keep your body straight, lean forward and slowly let your front knee bend. You will feel the stretch on the calf of your back leg. Your heel on the back leg should stay on the floor. Hold the stretch for 10 seconds. Repeat with your other leg.

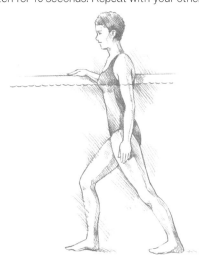

Your Workout: **Mix It Up**

When you start exercising, particularly if you have not exercised in a long time, you may not be able to do more than a little stretching and taking a walk. But as you progress to a higher stage of fitness, you can add more elements to your routine. Here, you'll learn how different activities fall into the three basic aspects of a complete exercise regimen.

FLEXIBILITY MOVEMENTS help maintain normal joint movement and relieve stiffness. In range-of-motion exercises, you do reaching and bending movements to move a joint as far as you comfortably can in every direction. A stretching routine before and after other physical activities also warms up and relaxes your muscles, reducing the chance of injury.
Activities: Stretching, yoga, tai chi, range-of-motion exercises such as shoulder shrugs, shoulder circles, arm reaches, arm circles.
Why do it? By keeping ligaments, tendons and joints flexible, you feel better and move easier.
How often? Can be done once or twice daily and should be done at least every other day.

AEROBIC OR ENDURANCE EXERCISE challenges the heart and lungs with continual movement as in walking, jogging, bicycling and swimming. Sustaining an elevated heart rate during each session improves cardiovascular and overall body fitness.
Activities: Walking, jogging or running, along with lower impact aerobic activities like bicycling (stationary or outdoor), aerobic dancing, ice skating, rowing (machine or outdoor) swimming and water aerobics.
Why do it? Aerobic exercise improves cardiovascular fitness, helps you sleep better, lifts your spirits and helps control weight. Studies have shown that cardiovascular exercise reduces your risk of heart disease, high blood pressure and some forms of cancer.
How often? Aerobic or endurance exercise should be done for 20 to 30 minutes three to five times a week.

STRENGTHENING EXERCISES also known as body sculpting or weight training, help maintain and increase your strength by working your muscles against some kind of resistance. Strength training helps strengthen the muscles around your joints to protect them from injury. It also helps you perform daily activities like climbing stairs.
Activities: Strength training includes many kinds of exercises, such as working out on weight machines, pulling against oversized rubber bands, doing isometric exercises (static exercises in which your joints don't move), using medicine balls, lifting free weights and resistance walking in water.
Why do it? Strong muscles help support and protect joints, make physical exertion easier and improve balance. Muscles that are strong also burn more calories.
How often? Can be done three times a week as long as you use light weights and should be done at least every other day. Proper form is essential.

SIDE LEG LIFT (HIP ABDUCTION AND ADDUCTION). Stand with your side to the pool wall, with your knees relaxed. Place your hand on the wall for balance. Swing your leg out to the side, toward the center of the pool and in toward the wall, crossing in front of your other leg. Repeat on the other side.

SIDE BEND (FLEXION). Place your hands on your hips with your feet shoulder-width apart and knees relaxed. Bend slowly to one side, with your hand sliding down your thigh as you bend. Return to starting position and bend to other side. Do not bend forward or twist or turn your trunk.

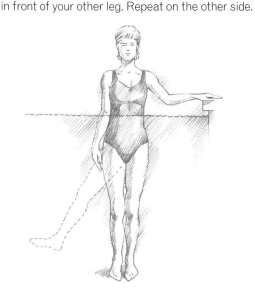

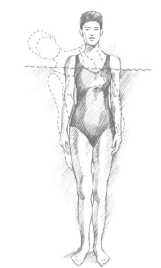

Guidelines for Strengthening Exercises

- Warm up before and cool down after exercising.
- Begin with one to two sets of five repetitions of each exercise. Gradually increase to three sets of eight reps of each exercise. If you can do more than eight reps, increase the weight until the last rep of each set if difficult.
- Perform the exercises without weight at first. If you decide to add weight, begin with weights of no more than one pound to three pounds.
- Do the same exercises for your left side and your right side.
- Do not hold your breath. Counting out loud ensures that you are not holding your breath.
- Strengthening exercises should be done three times a week. More is not necessarily better.
- If you experience any new or increased pain more than two hours after you exercise, you have done too much. First decrease the weight and then the number of repetitions.
- If you have had an injury or surgery on any part of your body or if you have a history of heart problems, consult your doctor before performing these exercises.
- Stop before you get tired. Muscle fatigue can result in increased strain on the joints and increased pain. By resting, you can increase your body's endurance.

You're on the Road to Fitness!

Whew! You've learned a lot about exercise and how it can benefit your efforts to change your life. In many ways, exercise is the most important aspect of achieving better health and fitness. You have some strategies for setting goals for getting some regular exercise, and you also have a variety of suggestions for fun, realistic exercise options you can try now.

As you discovered, staying motivated to exercise consistently is the most important aspect of getting fit. If you don't keep it up, your body's state of fitness won't improve. To stay motivated, you have to have a positive outlook on what you are trying to accomplish. As we learned in previous chapters, stress, anxiety or tension may cause people to get into a rut of bad health habits: eating unhealthy "comfort foods," avoiding exercise, feeling bad about yourself, losing a hopeful vision of your future.

Exercise can help you work out your stress and tension in a positive, healthy way. Improving your diet and losing excess pounds can be an uplifting enterprise. But getting to the root of your stress, and finding healthy ways to deal with it, is essential to making your inner and outer self healthier. If you are going to change your life, you have to improve your outlook on the road ahead. In the following chapter, we'll learn how stress may be affecting you and how you can get a grip on it!

CHANGE
YOUR
OUTLOOK

Improving the way you handle stress can make it easier for you to attain all of your other change-your-life goals.

Why is stress such a common word in our conversations today? You have probably either said or heard someone else say one of the following:

"I'm so stressed out."

"I can't believe I was so irritable today when somebody asked me about my relationship with my mother-in-law. It must just be stress."

"Work is causing me so much stress, I can't stop going to the snack machine."

"I hear my husband grind his teeth at night because he is so stressed out over his mother's illness. I can't sleep at night."

What Is Stress?

Stress. Why is this word mentioned so often in our daily conversations, often as the root of a million different problems or as the unwelcome result of problems? What is stress and why does

it affect our lives so much?

Stress refers to how the body reacts to situations that are upsetting, exciting, dangerous or annoying. Your reactions to stress can be both physical and mental.

Physical stress reactions can include sweating, increased body temperature, headaches, stomachaches, sleeplessness, tightened jaw or jaw pain, and increased heart rate. Mental reactions to stress can include worry, anxiety, tension, nightmares or angry outbursts. Often, you experience both physical and mental reactions to stress.

Stress is normal. Many situations in our lives can cause stress, such as a move to a new house, getting a new job or divorcing your spouse. Stressful events aren't always negative. A wedding is a happy occasion, but it can also be stressful. Ask anyone who has planned one!

If you're like most people, dealing with your stress is a daily challenge. What day goes by when

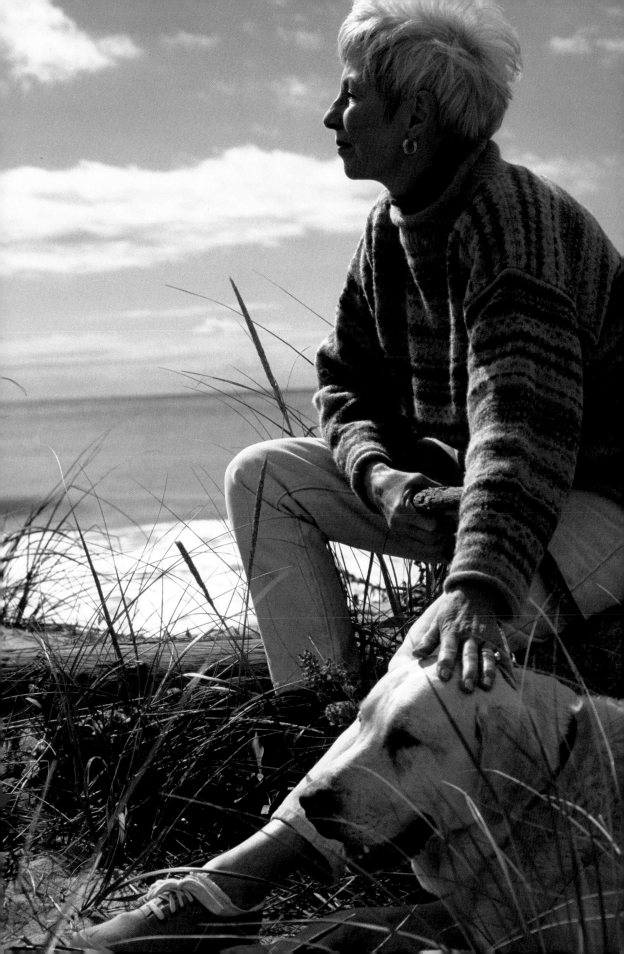

you don't experience some type of stress? Just getting in the car and driving to work can be stressful. Getting your kids dressed in the morning and ready to go to school can be stressful. Facing an important business meeting with a new client can be stressful. Even figuring out what shoes to wear with your new suit can be stressful!

But by learning simple strategies to ease or control your stress, you can reduce your stress reactions, feel healthier and manage your activities more effectively.

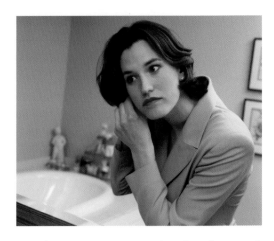

Putting It All in Perspective:
Positive Stress Vs. Negative Stress

Stress should be a temporary response, a sort of "emergency setting" for your body when faced with an important decision or situation. Stress revs your internal engines and shifts you into high gear, like when you pump on the gas pedal of your car.

Stress delivers an extra dose of a hormone called adrenaline to the rest of your body, temporarily increasing your blood pressure and heart rate and enabling you to cope with difficult situations. But if you get stuck on that revved-up setting, stress becomes unhealthy. Here are some differences between positive/healthy and negative/unhealthy stress reactions.

Healthy stress is followed by relaxation. Your mind and body balance your perceived demands. After you've handled the difficult or important situation, your body returns to its pre-stressed state – heartbeat and breathing slow, blood pressure goes down, muscles relax and so forth. Your physical and emotional energies recharge, so that you can meet the next challenge when it comes along.

Unhealthy stress occurs when the demands you perceive are greater than the physical and mental resources you perceive. In other words, you feel that the cause of your stress may be more than you can handle. So you stay "revved up" and don't relax.

Even after the source of this unhealthy stress goes away, your body remains in a stressed state. Your blood pressure and heart rate stay above normal, your stomach and muscles still feel tight. Because you don't relax, your body and mind are unable to recover energy and balance, so the next challenge is difficult to meet.

If you experience unhealthy stress on a regular basis, your stress becomes chronic, or long-lasting. With each additional challenge because your physical and emotional resources become more exhausted. Chronic stress can cause many negative effects on your body and mind, including:

- Headaches
- Stomach distress, ulcers
- High blood pressure
- Muscle tension, back pain and other types of pain
- Chronic fatigue
- Restlessness, irritability, frustration
- Decreased zest for life, worry, fear, depression
- Difficulty making decisions, forgetfulness

- Increased use of alcohol, cigarettes or drugs
- Eating and sleeping problems
- Disease or pain flares
- Poorer immune function

How Your Body Reacts to Stress

During stress, your body tenses. This muscle tension can cause pain or fatigue. This pain and fatigue (caused by stress-related sleeplessness, perhaps) can limit your abilities to do your everyday activities, not to mention special activities, making you feel frustrated and overwhelmed. This feeling, in turn, can cause you to become depressed. You don't exercise and you don't eat properly, causing your overall health to deteriorate.

What you have is a vicious cycle, a cycle of stress, pain, limited and lost abilities, depression and poor health. But if you understand how your body reacts physically and emotionally to stress and learn how to manage stress, you can help break that destructive cycle.

Consider these steps for controlling your stress:
- Identify the physical and emotional signs of stress.
- Identify the causes of your stress.
- Modify or eliminate the causes of your stress, or learn to handle them more effectively.

IDENTIFY YOUR PHYSICAL REACTIONS TO STRESS

You probably know how your body reacts to stress. During stress, the body quickly releases a chemical called epinephrine into your bloodstream. This process sets into motion a series of changes called the fight-or-flight response. Your heart beats faster, your breathing rate increases, your blood pressure rises and your muscles feel tense. Why does all this happen?

These physical changes are your body's natural way to give you added strength and energy to face the stressful event: giving a speech, meeting your new in-laws, dropping off your daughter at college. When stress is handled in a positive way, the body restores itself to a normal state.

At times, it may feel impossible to handle stress in a positive way. When this happens, stress-related tension builds like steam in a kettle. With no outlet, this tension (like steam) takes its toll on your body. It needs to be released. Unreleased tension can cause headaches, upset stomach, jaw pain and other problems.

IDENTIFY YOUR EMOTIONAL REACTIONS TO STRESS

How your mind reacts to stress is harder to predict than how your body reacts to stress. Emotional reactions are different from person to person and from stressful situation to situation. You might experience feelings of anxiety, fear, helplessness, anger, loss of control, frustration or annoyance.

A little stress can be a good thing – it can help you perform your best in an important situation, such as during an athletic event, a work presentation or during your community theater production. If you experience too much stress, though, you may make errors, become clumsy or get angry.

As we said earlier, your reactions to will not be the same as other people's reactions. Each person responds to stress differently. One person's stress may cause headaches, while another person gets an upset stomach.

Stress symptoms may be obvious or hard to identify. For example, you may assume that your upset stomach was caused by something you ate – until you notice the same thing happens every time you confront a stressful situation. Pay attention to your body's signals so you can learn how stress affects you personally.

In the box on this page, you will see some common reactions to stress. If you experience these without understanding the cause, they could be a reaction to stress in your life.

IDENTIFYING WHAT CAUSES YOUR STRESS

If you experience any of the physical or emotional reactions to stress in the box on this page, treating these problems with over-the-counter medications (antacid tablets, headache medication, topical analgesic creams for muscle aches) may help you feel better temporarily. These treatments will help alleviate your symptoms, but they won't address the cause of the symptoms. That's because the cause of the physical or emotional symptom you are experiencing is stress, not a virus, a spicy meal or your allergies.

Pay Attention to Your Body's Signals

The following physical and emotional reactions could mean stress. Do you ever experience these on a regular basis?

- headaches
- stomach upset or pains
- constipation or diarrhea
- uncontrollable crying
- sleeping problems, such as inability to fall asleep or oversleeping
- disturbing dreams
- tense muscles of shoulder, neck or back
- jaw pain
- grinding or clenching teeth at night
- loss of appetite
- general anxiety, such as moodiness, anger, worry
- poor concentration
- cold, clammy hands
- dry mouth

You need to discover the underlying cause of your stress if you are going to "treat" the problem. If you learn the sources of your stress, you can predict a stressful situation before it happens and deal with it more effectively when it does happen.

Think about what is going on in your life right now. What causes you the most stress, anxiety, worry or concern? What situations make you nervous or fearful? Meeting new people? Talking to your boss? Seeing your family? Trying new things? Once you know what things cause you to become stressed, you can set goals on how to change these things or adapt to them.

Keeping a Stress Diary

As with challenges related to diet or exercise, keeping a written record of what causes you stress can be a great way to conquer stress. You can use your Changes Journal to record events in your life that cause stress, as well as any physical or emotional symptoms that occur with these events.

When you do your weekly review, look for patterns in your stress reaction symptoms. You will probably be able to figure out what causes these reactions and make adjustments. You will not be able to avoid every stressful situation – even if you move into a cave! But you can avoid some situations and be prepared for the others.

Seeing patterns in your journal will show you that board meetings make you stressed out. So find a way to relax before your next board meeting (we'll give you strategies in this chap-

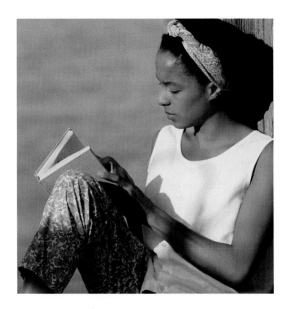

It might feel weird to write down the causes of your stress or how you react. That isn't as easy as writing down how far you walked or what you ate for dinner. But once you learn to recognize what is really causing your stress, and linking this stress to particular reactions, you'll find it easier. Below is an example.

Changing or Dealing With the Causes of Your Stress

Once you've discovered what causes your stress, determine which stressful situations can be changed – and which are here for good. You can only change what you can control. Here are some simple strategies that may help:

Set goals concerning stress control and develop a plan of action for reaching them. Can you delegate some responsibilities to friends or family members? Can you have some flexibility about when you finish a household task or a project at work? Can you say no to friends who ask you to do more than you think you can handle?

List your priorities. What do you have to do right now? What can you do later? What can you eliminate? For example, you may have to

ter). Learn how to say "no" to certain stressful activities that may be unnecessary.

As we have learned, an important first step to eliminating stress is to identify what causes it and how you respond both physically and emotionally. By using your Changes Journal to record what events cause your stress and how you react to it, you should start to discover a pattern of stressors and symptoms. Once you determine what things, people, events or situations "stress you out," then you can become more prepared for dealing with stress using some of the techniques in this book.

SAMPLE STRESS JOURNAL

Date	Time	Cause of Stress	Physical Symptoms	Emotional Symptoms
4/18	7 a.m.	Getting kids on school bus on time	Fast heartbeat, tight jaw	feel rushed, disorganized
4/18	8 a.m.	Stuck in traffic	heartbeat races, clammy palms	frustrated, angry at being late
4/18	9 a.m.	Meeting with new client	stomach fluttery, dry throat, headache later	anxious, nervous

bake a cake for the neighborhood fundraiser tonight, but can you put off doing your laundry until Tuesday?

Reduce hassles. If rush hour commuting bothers you, consider taking public transportation or map out a new way to drive to work – a longer one, if necessary – to avoid high-traffic areas. If certain people, situations or places annoy you, avoid them if you can. Don't go to the mall during the holiday shopping season if the crowds get on your nerves. Shop online, through catalogs or at individual stores outside the mall.

Set a goal to increase your uplifting activities and decrease your aggravating ones. Take some time to list in your journal which activities lift your spirits and which ones drag you down. Compare the two lists. Can you give up some aggravating activities so you'll have more time to do the things you like?

When making a decision about whether or not to do something, ask yourself, "Am I taking care of my needs also?" It's easy to become caught up in what others need or want at the expense of your own emotional health. It's not worth the expense.

Learn to say no without feeling guilty. You can decline to take part in activities if you feel that you can't handle any more tasks. It doesn't have to be a permanent change – if you find that later on you have less stress and more time, you can go back to doing something you gave up earlier, such as volunteer work.

As you have learned earlier in this book, changing your life means finding the right balance of what you want to do and what you need to do for your health. It's no different when it comes to your outlook. You can't do it all! But you know that you must do certain things and

have to find the right balance of obligations and pleasures to keep your stress level under control.

> ## "Am I taking care of my needs also?"

Seek solutions and compromises with others. If you and your spouse fight because one person wants to go to the movies on Saturday and the other person wants to watch football, maybe you can find a compromise. One weekend you can watch football together, and on another weekend (particularly if the game doesn't seem as "important"), you can go to the movies together. If the other people in your life aren't so willing to compromise, let them know that you are trying to seek a solution for your emotional health. At some point, you'll have to decide what is most important for your needs.

Learning To Say No

In our increasingly busy lives, having an overloaded schedule – what we often call "being overextended" – is a fact of life. You may find yourself taking on more and more responsibilities and feeling overwhelmed by the amount you have to do each week. What is the typical result of all these activities and obligations? Stress.

You may feel that you can't cut out the responsibilities, obligations and events crowding your life. Frankly, there are some things you cannot cut out. But there are some things you can turn down – not the things you really love to do, but things you may prefer not to do at all. It's OK to say "no" to some things. And it's OK to lose the guilt!

Turning down extra duties that are not necessary to your job, your health or your closest personal relationships can be healthy – this action can even temporarily reduce your stress. Why not give "no" a try? Here are some suggestions:

1. Practice saying "no" in front of the mirror. We're not kidding. Give it a try. Sit in front of the mirror when nobody is around, and say "no" out loud, five times. "No." It's not so difficult, is it?

2. Set goals for what you really want to get done. You can't do everything – that leads to stress and the accompanying physical and emotional problems that are making you miserable. So ask yourself: What do you really want to do? Is your family the highest priority? Perhaps being a spectator at your son's weekly soccer match is an important goal for you. Or attending church services at least one night each week is something you cherish.

List the things you really have to do – like work, taking care of yourself, chores – and the things you really want to do – like the soccer match or church. Sit down for a moment with your calendar. Develop a plan for achieving those important goals, a plan that includes fun activities, hobbies, family and friends. Perhaps you can cut certain activities out of your schedule, or only do them once in a while. You may be able to delegate some responsibilities to other people. Remember: If you always say "yes" to every request, people will continue to ask you to do everything! Try that little word again: "No."

3. Figure out your priorities. As we said earlier, ask yourself what is important to you and the smooth functioning of your daily life. What tasks need to be done immediately? What can be done later? What can be eliminated? You may need to buy meat for dinner today, but perhaps you can do laundry tomorrow. Decide what non-essential tasks and activities is a priority for you, and say "yes" to those things, "no" to others.

4. Say "no" to unnecessary hassles when you can. You may think that some sources of stress cannot be avoided or eliminated. Is that true? Look at the stressors again. If rush-hour commuting bothers you, could you figure out a new, more peaceful route to work? Is it possible to take public transportation on certain days? You may be able to avoid certain annoying people and places. If you know that you need your lunch hour for quiet time, say "no" to your friends' offer to dine out at a crowded, loud restaurant. Or spend every other lunch hour on your own – people will understand.

Judge what your peace of mind is worth to you. Mowing the lawn may be an energizing release for some people, but an unpleasant chore for others. Could you ask your son to mow the lawn, or offer to help him with some task in exchange for mowing the lawn? Consider hiring someone to mow the lawn, if the cost is worth it to you? Weigh your options and the cost of each one. Your health is worth a great deal.

5. Pamper yourself – it's a priority! Ask yourself: "Does this decision or action take care of, or work for, me?" You may find yourself in the role of everybody's caretaker. You say "yes" to every request because you feel that your family and friends depend on you. It's easy to take care of others at the expense of your own health. Say "no" to some requests, particularly those that you know others could handle. Take time to do things you enjoy. Earlier in this book, we asked you to make a list of things you love to do to

celebrate your everyday victories. Use some of the items you listed as a way to pamper yourself when you are feeling stressed.

6. Think "win/win." When figuring out a plan of action, seek solutions that will benefit everybody. If you want to go for a walk, and your spouse has chores to do, help finish the work and go walking together. You will enjoy the time you spend together walking, and you will know that the necessary chores were completed. Teamwork can ease the burden for everyone.

You can only change yourself, not other people. Some situations can't be changed, but you can modify your point of view. There is an old expression: "Roll with the punches." You need to be flexible in order to keep stress under control. Being flexible helps you keep a positive attitude, despite problems or conflicts that arise. You can say "no" to unnecessary obligations or activities, but you know that at times, you have to agree to do things that stress you out. Remember that these duties won't last forever. Keep the joyful events on your calendar in mind to get you through the stressful times.

You Can't Change Situations, But You Can Change Your Outlook

The only things you can change are the things you can control. That is the one firm rule of life. You can change how you behave and you react, but you can't change how other people behave and react.

Many situations can't be changed. If your job causes you stress, you may have to realize that your job won't change, but your point of view can. Try to be flexible and develop a positive attitude despite hardships. Here are some ways to help you change your outlook.

Think positively. Ask yourself if a stressful situation has any benefit that you can't see at first. Getting laid off from your job could lead to a spiral of depression, debts and debilitating pain. Or it could be an opportunity to change your work situation for the better and get into a new career path that is more to your liking.

Do a reality check. Evaluate the stressful situation's real importance. Your boss didn't say anything to you after your presentation. Does that mean he didn't like your presentation or didn't have anything to criticize you about? Or was he busy and distracted by his own projects? If you didn't get outright criticism, perhaps it's not as earth-shattering as you thought it was.

Develop support systems. Share your feelings of stress or anxiety with family, friends, counselors, clergy or others who are good listeners. Sharing can help you view problems constructively. Try not to whine constantly about every detail of your discomfort. You might turn everyone off and make people wary of listening to you when you really need help.

Put things in perspective. When you feel anxiety about your life, think about something or someone else – your sister, your neighbor, the last movie you saw – to distract you and help you relax.

Develop "safety valves." Release your stress positively by letting it out. Exercise, do something fun or write in your journal to process your feelings and get in touch with what is bothering you.

Relaxing To Reduce Symptoms of Stress

Relaxing is one of the best ways to cope with stress. Relaxation means more than just sitting on the couch with the TV on. It is a serious, active process, requiring practice, to calm your body and mind.

Remember, stress has many causes, which means there are many solutions. You need to understand not only what is causing your stress, but what methods will really help you control your stress. Everyone will not find the same strategies helpful. Whatever works for you is what's important. Try different strategies until you find something that works well to relieve your anxiety and stress.

If you find that your stress is getting out of control or you are having trouble finding ways to relax, you may wish to see a mental-health professional or consult your doctor. If stress is causing you to have chronic physical or emotional symptoms, a health-care professional will be able to either prescribe medications to help you control anxiety or suggest ways you can control your stress. This person can also listen to your feelings and help you identify the causes of your problems.

There are some great methods for relaxation. Your doctor or any mental-health professional can recommend a strategy that is right for your needs, but you can also find activities or methods on your own. These activities should help you work out your frustration or anger positively, or help you unwind and "relax" tense muscles and a tight stomach. They should be things you enjoy doing, not activities that increase your feeling of obligation, duty or aggravation.

Some of these activities might include:

- Taking a warm bath with some of your favorite soothing music playing on the stereo
- Hitting golf balls at the driving range for an hour

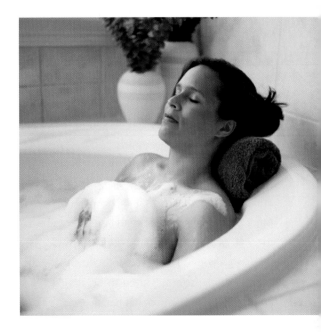

- Taking a brisk walk in the park
- Doing volunteer work
- Doing a yoga (an exercise and relaxation practice developed in ancient India) routine with a videotape or at a yoga class
- Meditation or prayer
- Organizing your old photographs into albums
- Dancing to your favorite oldies in your basement or living room

Get Real!

Do a reality check during stressful situations by asking yourself these questions:
- Does this situation reflect a threat by signaling harm, or a challenge by signaling an opportunity?
- Are there other ways to look at this situation?
- What exactly is at stake?
- What is the worst that can happen?
- What are you afraid will occur?
- What evidence do you have that this will happen?
- Is there evidence that contradicts this conclusion?
- What coping resources are available?

- Being with friends or loved ones who lift your spirits
- Gardening or yardwork

Depending on your personal feelings, relaxation might be something you can do with others or on your own. See what works for you. If you find that when you are stressed you feel better when you get away from other people, then use relaxation strategies that don't involve others. At times, other people – even friends and family – can be the external pressures that cause your stress. Or, they may cause you to be "keyed up" when you really need to relax. You may need to be alone to find your own sense of emotional balance.

Here are some very specific strategies for relaxing your body and mind. Try these at a time when you experience stress, or possible physical or emotional reactions to stress. Note the results. If a practice works well to relieve your stress, use it again! If at any time, you feel dizzy or light-headed, stop the practice.

DEEP BREATHING

To practice deep breathing, sit in a comfortable chair with your feet on the floor and your arms at your sides. Close your eyes and breathe in deeply, saying to yourself , "I am….," then exhale slowly saying, "…relaxed."

Continue to breathe slowly, silently repeating something to yourself such as, "My hands are warm, my feet are warm, my breathing is deep and smooth, my heartbeat is calm and steady. I feel calm and at peace."

GUIDED IMAGERY

Guided imagery also helps you distract yourself from what may be causing your stress. It's an easy, safe and free way to unwind and release tension.

To practice guided imagery, do the following:
- Close your eyes, take a deep breath and hold in for several seconds.
- Breathe out slowly, feeling your body relax as you do.
- Now, think about a place where you have been where you felt safe and comfortable. It could be in your childhood home, at the beach, at your favorite mountain hideaway or at your summer camp.
- Imagine this place in as much detail as possible. Imagine the sounds you heard – of waves against the sand, seagulls calling overhead, children laughing on the beach. Imagine the way it felt, smelled and tasted – the salt water on your lips, the soft sand beneath your feet, the ocean breeze blowing through your hair.
- Try to remember and recapture the positive feelings you had when you were there.
- Keep these feelings, sensations and thoughts in your mind.
- Take several more deep breaths.
- Enjoy feeling calm and peaceful for five more minutes.
- Now, open your eyes.

PROGRESSIVE RELAXATION

Progressive relaxation is a strategy in which you progressively tense and then relax all of your body's muscles, from head to toe.

To practice progressive relaxation, do the following:
- Close your eyes.
- Take a deep breath, expanding your lungs and breathing all the way down to your gut.
- Breathe out, and feel your stress flow out with your breath.

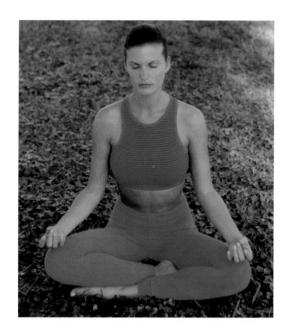

- Starting with your feet and calves, slowly tense your muscles.
- Hold for several seconds, then release and relax these muscles.
- Slowly, using the same technique, work your way through up your body: thighs and buttocks, back and stomach muscles, hands and arms, shoulders and neck, until you have tensed and relaxed the muscles of your neck and face.
- Continue breathing, quietly, for a few minutes.
- Enjoy the feeling of relaxation.
- Now, open your eyes.

Moving Ahead:
Changing Your Outlook for Good

Now you have some important information on why you may be experiencing stress, what physical and emotional reactions you may be experiencing due to your stress, how to identify what is causing you stress and what you can do to release that stress in a healthy, positive way. What's the next step?

It's important to set some goals in this area also, because although you may not experience stress every day (or maybe you do), outlook improvement is something you should strive for every day.

With a positive outlook, you will be able to move forward with your other goals related to diet and exercise. If your outlook is negative, you won't feel motivated to keep your diet healthy and to get your physical activity. By reading this book, you have learned that stress, anxiety, tension and frustration are often the root cause of why we eat poorly or too much, and why we sit on the couch instead of getting up and exercising.

Stress is an increasingly common problem in our fast-paced society, when our environments change from day to day. You may be able to acclimate yourself to one stressful change, but then something else comes along to make your stress level rise again. Following are some steps to put stress in the back seat and develop a more positive outlook.

STEP ONE:

Figure Out What Causes Your Stress

As we learned earlier, you need to identify the effects of stress on your physical and emotional states. Realize that you can't change everything in your life that may cause your stress. You may not be able to quit your job or give your kids to someone else. But you can change the way you react to the stress in your life. You can control your outlook.

STEP TWO:

Look at Your Stressor in a Different Way

You might admire how your coworker reacts to stressful situations at the office, staying calm when you are breaking into a sweat over the monthly sales figures. Your friend's calm exterior doesn't mean he or she isn't experiencing stress – but he or she handles it in a better way.

Are there people you know who seem to handle difficult situations well? Think about the people you admire, who seem to "take things in stride." You can even think about people you knew in the past, such as a teacher or a mentor, or even people you don't know well but admire from a distance, such as a public figure.

How does this person react to adversity? List the strengths and positive stress-control techniques that this person seems to have. For example, you may react to a difficult question from your boss by getting nervous and answering quickly off the top of your head. But you notice that your coworker, in the same situation, takes a deep breath, ponders the question and answers slowly and reasonably, or says, "I don't know about that, but I can find out."

Now, which of this person's strengths relate to you? Which techniques could you try to emulate? Did you have an aunt who lost her husband in wartime, leaving her to raise her kids alone? Did she manage to remain optimistic about life, despite the fact that she experienced a personal tragedy and had to take on more responsibility than she expected? Could you emulate her attitude and apply it to your own problems?

STEP THREE

Make a Positive Plan for Dealing With Stress.

Are you angry when you are experiencing stress? Of course you are. You build up anger and you don't know how to let it go. You may be angry at a person who seems to be causing you stress, such as your spouse, your boss, your mother, your best friend. Or you may be angry at a situation, such as the economy, or even

angry with yourself for the way you react to stressful situations.

Do you react to stressful situations the same way that you did when you were a child? Did you learn these reactions by watching your family? Did your family deal with anger or stress by staying silent, bottling the feelings inside and never letting them out? Or did they scream insults at each other? Did people in your family deal with their negative feelings by negative behaviors such as alcohol use, drug use or binge eating?

How your family dealt with anger, stress and tension is a big part of how you deal with the same issues. Your family's behavior probably molded your behavior. These reactions to stress are the coping techniques you learned as a child, so you carry them with you as an adult. And for many people, these lifelong techniques don't work!

You have to let these old techniques go. They are hurting you rather than helping you. You need to find a new way to deal with stressful events. Those bad habits and negative reactions are only hurting you and the people around you. You have been saying the same things to yourself repeatedly, and these words hurt you and hold you back from having a positive outlook on life.

You need to identify a new way to react to stress. If you keep things inside, find a way to let them out! Write in your journal or talk to a friend or counselor. If you find that you scream at your spouse when you are upset about something at work, learn to not shift the blame onto an innocent party. Talk to your spouse instead, and see if you can find solutions to your problems at work.

STEP FOUR

Make a Contract With Yourself
To Deal With Stress in a Healthy Way.

You can use the contract form in Chapter

Two, just as you did for your diet and exercise goals. Identify some strategies, using our suggestions, for releasing stress and finding relaxation. You will wish to set some general goals for how you will work relaxation techniques like the ones described above into your regular routine. For example, you might contract to try guided imagery or deep breathing exercises three times a week after work. Incorporating these activities (which may only take a few minutes to do) into your regular routine may help you keep stress levels down. You could also contract with yourself to try a relaxation activity right after a stressful event.

Or, you may wish to create a separate, simpler goal sheet where you identify the causes of your stress, your typical reaction (which is unhealthy) and a new technique (which is healthy). Here's how:

1. Take a fresh piece of paper and write three headings across the top. The first heading should be "Cause of Stress." Below this heading, list some of the common stressors in your life that you identified earlier in this chapter. For example, you might list "talking to my mother-in-law each week."

2. The second heading should be "How I Usually React." Next to the entry "talking to my mother-in-law each week," you might write, "holding anger inside; screaming at husband afterward."

3. The third heading should be "Better Ways to React." In this column, you will list a few suggestions (like those we discussed earlier) for more healthy ways you could handle this stressful situation. For example, you might write, "try to breathe; keep conversation to no more than five minutes; play soft music in the background."

This goal sheet is a way for you to identify what causes your stress, recognize the unhealthy way you react to stress and strategize healthier ways to deal with stress.

DEVELOP A SUPPORT NETWORK

Locate a support network of friends you can lean on, people you can talk to when you experience stress or anxiety, or who will join you for fun, uplifting activities when you need to release tension.

Most people know what they need to do to get their stress under control. But it's hard to do it. It's much easier to fall into old, negative habits. It might help you to have someone who can help you, motivate you and encourage you to make these changes.

Make an agreement with your friend that he or she will be there for you in times of great stress. Agree to help your friend when he or she need a stress release in return. Develop a short list of people you can turn to when you need to

SAMPLE STRESS GOAL SHEET

Cause of Stress	How I Usually React	Better Ways To React
Customer call	Biting nails	Deep breathing exercise

talk or vent during times of anxiety, stress, fear or tension. Ask these people, "Can I call you sometime if I really need some help or advice?"

Having several people will make it easier for you to have someone available when you really need it. Plus, you won't be turning to the same person all the time! Agree to listen to them when they have built-up feelings of stress and tension.

You can change your outlook and find new ways to deal with stress and anxiety. You don't

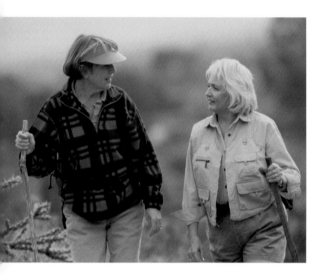

have to fall into the same trap over and over again. You have to be prepared to let go of the negative experiences of the past – don't feel bitter about what happened a long time ago. You need to embrace the future and feel that today is

the first step in a new journey toward a healthier, happier you.

EMBRACE THE JOY OF NOW

What is fulfilling in your life right now? You may think that your life is stressful, boring and hopeless. But there must be joyful things in your life – your children, your loved ones, your friends and your accomplishments. Take note of these things and appreciate them. Reward yourself when something good happens so you don't let the positive times slip by unnoticed. You spend plenty of time focusing on the negative aspects of life; why not focus on the uplifting things too?

As you can see, changing your life means changing how you feel physically and how you feel emotionally. Changing your life means changing the way you react to situations in your life – and how you act as you go through your life. Change is a gradual process. You won't suddenly become stress-free! People, events and circumstances will still cause stress in your life. But you can work to change the way you feel about yourself and your life. You can do it gradually, just as you make gradual changes to your diet and fitness to make the improvements stick. You can change. By taking the step to read this book and try some of the exercises or techniques offered, you already have.

NOW IS THE TIME TO CHANGE YOUR LIFE

Now that you've learned the three aspects of change and some great techniques for making permanent, positive change, get going!

Each of the three aspects of change is connected to each other. Each is a point on a circle that cannot be broken. Think of this circle as a flow of energy. Your diet, your fitness and your outlook are each stations along this energy flow. If one of the stations falters, the energy cannot flow properly and the other stations cannot function.

If you experience chronic, negative reactions to stress, you are less likely to exercise and eat right. If you don't exercise and eat right, you won't feel very good physically, causing you to be emotionally "down" and not giving your body the energy it needs to handle stress positively. When your life is in balance, the energy along that circle is flowing properly. Everything works better!

We hope you have found some useful strategies in this book for making that energy flow properly. We have offered you some simple ideas that you can incorporate into your life right now.

Be patient with yourself. Progress may come slowly. But it will come. Don't be discouraged if you don't see a drastic change in yourself right away. You need to stay committed to the positive changes you make, because they will make a big difference in the way you feel. So change your life and don't give up! Be realistic about the first steps you will take. Once you incorporate a few changes in your life, you will find that it's much easier to take them to the next level. You can accomplish what you have dreamed of if you just take it one small step at a time.

Everyone, no matter what stage they are in now, has goals for the future. They aspire to improve something in their life, whether it is their physical fitness, their diet or their emotional outlook. The way to change your life for the better is to identify what you need to change, set goals for making that change, pick some first steps, and then get started on those steps. You can make a contract with yourself, specifically identifying things you can and will do to make that change happen. You can rely on friends and family, if you need to, to give you motivation and support when you find that you're slipping on your goals. You can seek professional help if you need it for concrete guidance.

THE MISSION OF THE ARTHRITIS FOUNDATION

This book was published by the Arthritis Foundation, the only national, not-for-profit health agency serving the more than 43 million Americans with some form of arthritis. The mission of the Arthritis Foundation is to improve lives through leadership in the prevention, control and cure of arthritis and related diseases.

In addition to this book, the Arthritis Foundation has many resources to help in your quest to improve yourself and change your life. The Arthritis Foundation has a great deal of information for people who may be at risk for developing this serious disease – millions of Americans fall into this category. By getting your weight under control and being more physically active, you may be able to prevent arthritis, or at least you can lessen its impact if you do develop arthritis later in life. The steps you take now will make your life so much healthier and happier later on. We can help!

To find your local chapter of the Arthritis Foundation, call 800/283-7800 or log on to www.arthritis.org. The Web site features a great deal of free information about health, fitness and wellness, including brochures and an interactive program called *Connect and Control*, where you can input your personal health information and see what steps you should take to improve your health. You can read current and past issues of *Arthritis Today*, the magazine that inspired this book. *Arthritis Today* has a wealth of information on arthritis, but also on general health, fitness and wellness issues important to everyone. You can subscribe by calling 800/207-8633 or on the Web site.

The Arthritis Foundation also sells a variety of books and videos to offer you more information on health issues and to stay fit and active, no matter what your current physical state. The Foundation supports research on preventing and curing arthritis and related diseases, and you can find out more about ways you can participate in and help with these efforts.

Most of all, the Arthritis Foundation is here to support your efforts to get healthy, stay healthy and become more active. We hope you have enjoyed this book. Use it to spur your efforts to lose weight, get fit and improve your outlook. Enjoy your future!

Your CHANGES JOURNAL

Photocopy this sample journal to use to track your daily actions, successes and challenges. Or, set up your own journal in a blank book or calendar book.

Basic Goals for Changing My Life:

Diet:

1. _____

_____

2. _____

_____

3. _____

_____

Exercise:

1. _____

_____

2. _____

_____

3. _____

_____

Outlook:

1. _____

_____

2. _____

_____

3. _____

_____

Change Your Life!
CHANGES JOURNAL

date:

SUNDAY

	Diet	Exercise	Outlook
morning			
midday			
evening			
late night			

challenges

triumphs

Change Your Life!
CHANGES JOURNAL

date:

_____

MONDAY

	Diet	Exercise	Outlook
morning			
midday			
evening			
late night			

challenges

_____

triumphs

_____

Change Your Life!
CHANGES JOURNAL

date:

TUESDAY

	Diet	Exercise	Outlook
morning			
midday			
evening			
late night			

challenges

triumphs

Change Your Life!
CHANGES JOURNAL

date:

WEDNESDAY

	Diet	Exercise	Outlook
morning			
midday			
evening			
late night			

challenges

triumphs

Change Your Life!
CHANGES JOURNAL

date:

THURSDAY

	Diet	Exercise	Outlook
morning			
midday			
evening			
late night			

challenges

triumphs

Change Your Life!
CHANGES JOURNAL

date:

FRIDAY

	Diet	Exercise	Outlook
morning			
midday			
evening			
late night			

challenges

triumphs

Change Your Life!
CHANGES JOURNAL

date:

SATURDAY

	Diet	Exercise	Outlook
morning			
midday			
evening			
late night			

challenges

triumphs

weight:

Resources for Good Living

The Arthritis Foundation, the only national, voluntary health organization that works for the more than 43 million Americans with arthritis or related diseases, offers many valuable resources through more than 150 offices nationwide. The chapter that serves your area has information, products, classes and other services to help you take control of your arthritis or related condition. To find the chapter nearest you, call 800/283-7800 or search the Arthritis Foundation Web site at www.arthritis.org.

Programs and Services

- Physician referral – Most Arthritis Foundation chapters can provide a list of doctors in your area who specialize in the evaluation and treatment of arthritis and arthritis-related diseases.

- Exercise programs – The Arthritis Foundation sponsors, develops and coordinates exercise programs for people with arthritis, featuring specially-trained instructors. They include:

- Walk With Ease – This course allows participants to develop a walking plan that meets their individual needs, accompanied by the Arthritis Foundation book Walk With Ease: Your Guide to Walking for Better Health, Improved Fitness and Less Pain. A program leader's manual is also available for those interested in participating in a group format.

- PACE (People with Arthritis Can Exercise) – These courses feature gentle movements to increase joint flexibility, range of motion, stamina and muscle strength. An accompanying video is available for home use.

- Arthritis Foundation Aquatic Program – These water exercise programs help relieve strain on muscles and joints. An accompanying PEP (Pool Exercise Program) video is available for home use.

- Self-Help Courses – The Arthritis Foundation sponsors mutual-support groups that provide opportunities for discussion and problem-solving among people with arthritis. In addition, the Arthritis Foundation offers courses designed to help people actively manage their particular disease through exercise, medications, relaxation techniques, pain management, nutrition and more. These are the Fibromyalgia Self-Help Course and the Arthritis Self-Help Course.

Information and Products

Find the latest information about arthritis, including research, medications, government advocacy, programs and services through one of the many information resources offered by the Arthritis Foundation:

- www.arthritis.org – Information about arthritis is available 24 hours a day on the Internet at the Arthritis Foundation's interactive, comprehensive Web site. Find news about arthritis, ways to get involved, and a variety of useful arthritis products, including books, brochures, videos and more. In addition, the Arthritis Foundation has a new interactive self-management guide for people with arthritis, Connect and Control: Your Online Arthritis Action Guide. Via questionnaire responses, Connect and Control helps participants create a customized management program for their unique situation.

- Arthritis Answers – Call toll-free at 800/283-7800 for 24-hour, automated information about arthritis and Arthritis Foundation resources. Trained volunteers and staff are also available at your local Arthritis Foundation chapter to answer questions or refer you to physicians and other resources. For general questions about arthritis, you can also call 404/872-7100 ext. 1, or e-mail questions to help@arthritis.org.

Publications

The Arthritis Foundation offers many publications to educate people with arthritis, as well as their families and friends, about diagnosis, medications, exercise, diet, pain management and more.

- Books – The Arthritis Foundation publishes a variety of books on arthritis to help you learn to understand and manage your condition, live a healthier life, and cope with the emotional challenges that come with a chronic illness. Order books at www.arthritis.org or by calling 800/207-8633. All Arthritis Foundation books are also available at your local bookstore.

- Brochures – The Arthritis Foundation offers brochures containing concise, understandable information on the many arthritis-related diseases and conditions. Topics include surgery, the latest medications, guidance for working with your doctors and self-managing your illness. Single copies are available free of charge at www.arthritis.org or by calling 800/283-7800.

- *Arthritis Today* – This award-winning bimonthly magazine provides the latest information on research, new treatments, trends and tips from experts and readers to help you manage arthritis. A one-year subscription to *Arthritis Today* is included when you become a member of the Arthritis Foundation. Annual membership is $20 and helps fund research to find cures for arthritis. Call 800/933-0032 for information.

- *Kids Get Arthritis Too* – This newsletter focusing on juvenile rheumatic diseases is published six times a year. Features speak to children and teens with the illness as well as to their parents. Stories examine the latest news in diagnosis, treatment and research of children's rheumatic diseases, as well as helpful ways kids can cope with their illnesses and the challenges they bring. This newsletter is now a benefit of membership in the Arthritis Foundation for people affected by juvenile rheumatic diseases. For information, call 800/283-7800.

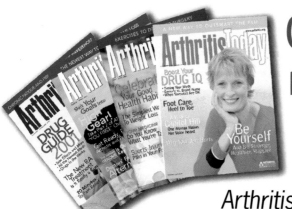

Get *Arthritis Today* magazine!

Now there are TWO ways to begin receiving the award-winning *Arthritis Today* magazine.

1 Become a member and get *Arthritis Today*, plus much more!

Become an Arthritis Foundation Member and receive a year (6 issues) of *Arthritis Today* – delivered to your home every-other month! Plus, you'll get all of these benefits...

- The 22-page **Drug Guide**, packed with information on hundreds of medications, their side effects and more.

- Personalized **Membership Card** with your special **Member Identification number**.

- **Members-only 10% discount** on all Foundation books and video purchases

- **Special announcements** about self-help and education programs.

- Access to the **Arthritis Specialists Referral List**.

- **Special updates** on cutting-edge arthritis research.

- **Invitations** to regional and local events and programs.

- By request, a **BONUS** subscription to *Kids Get Arthritis Too,* a bi-monthly newsletter filled with information to help families with arthritis.

You get all this for a minimum donation of $20.00! And most importantly, your tax-deductible membership donation will support critical arthritis research and community services.

Call your personal membership representative today!
1-800-933-0032

Membership dues are a minimum of twenty US dollars for twelve months, of which six dollars are designated for six issues of Arthritis Today. Your membership dues are tax deductible minus the six dollars allocated for the magazine.

22899704N

2 Subscribe to *Arthritis Today*!

Get the health magazine written just for you. In each information packed issue you'll find the latest on:

- **treatments**
- **research**
- **medications**
- **alternative therapies**
- **nutrition**
- **exercise**
- **and more!**

A year's subscription (6 issues) costs just $12.95, that's 45% off the newsstand price. Every issue of *Arthritis Today* contains information to help you live well. Get the tools you need to have an active healthy life!

Call the special subscription Hotline number
1-800-207-8633

21799792A

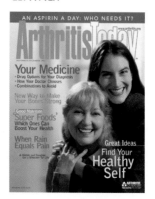

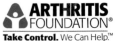